As an international executive coach and academic, working with and for prestigious global organisations, Dr Angélique du Toit spent much of her career supporting individuals and teams in their personal development. She is also an acclaimed author and contributor to the coaching profession. Drawing on her extensive experience as a coach and former fashion designer, Angélique now works with older women in her capacity as a coach and professional image consultant.

This book is dedicated to all H.A.G.S. around the world.

Angélique du Toit

H.A.G.S. WITH ATTITUDE: A PHILOSOPHY FOR AGEING

AUSTIN MACAULEY PUBLISHERS™
LONDON • CAMBRIDGE • NEW YORK • SHARJAH

A CIP catalogue record for this title is available from the British Library.

ISBN 9781398408685 (Paperback)
ISBN 9781398408692 (ePub e-book)

www.austinmacauley.com

First Published (2021)
Austin Macauley Publishers Ltd
25 Canada Square
Canary Wharf
London
E14 5LQ

I am enormously indebted to two inspiring ladies who generously took the time to review my book and provide some very valuable feedback and suggestions. They are Liz Clothier and Ruth Leggett. I am also grateful to my husband for his feedback and it was immensely valuable to get a different perspective and the viewpoint from a man's position. So many of the joys and challenges we face on the journey of getting older are shared by both males and females.

Introduction

'Be the kind of woman that when your feet hit the floor each morning, the devil says, "Oh crap, she's up!"'

– Unknown

This book is aimed at women who refuse to collude with society and the media, determined not to pass into insignificance having reached the magic age of 50 and beyond. My aim is to encourage and inspire women to be bold and to embrace this new phase of life with vigour, pursuing long lost dreams and indulging in guilt-free pursuits. We are never too old to have fun!

Just to be clear, this is not a self-help book and there are no 7, 10 or 20 steps you can follow to a blissfully happy life. Instead, it is more of practical philosophy, a way to make sense of and navigate the experiences of life beyond 50. It doesn't advocate a Pollyanna approach that everything will be hunky-dory if you merely chant the appropriate mantras. However, what this would do throughout is to encourage you to take responsibility for your life, irrespective of the challenges and yes, also opportunities that accompany life at this stage. So, the theme of the book is absolutely about attitude and philosophy for ageing well, happy and contented, whatever that may mean to you.

Throughout this book, I will challenge the anti-ageing attitude that seeps into every aspect of life. Instead, I will offer counter-arguments to support my fundamental disagreement with this prevailing rhetoric and associated beliefs. Moving beyond the paradigm of loss and decline is the growing popularity of successful ageing and what that entails. I will offer many arguments and research to support why this is critical to our physical as well as mental wellbeing as we get older.

Let's first of all address the issue of H.A.G.S. as the title. Why hags? How insulting! The reason is threefold. Firstly, to prevent us from taking life and ourselves too seriously; secondly, to understand the true meaning of hags and therefore as a metaphor for exploring the stories society and we tell ourselves in relation to women of a certain age and thirdly, as a pneumonic that captures the key themes of the book, namely:

H	Healthy living
A	Attitude
G	Get up and go
S	Social connections

Hags are powerful characters often dominating stories and fantasies, feared for their magical abilities. The stories we tell ourselves about our identities, as older women, are equally powerful in leading us down dark woods where dangers lurk. Instead, our magical powers can be of benefit to society as well as ourselves.

All of the research I have done for this book points to the importance of what the mnemonic represents. Embracing the wisdom of H.A.G.S. in every aspect will not only enhance the quality of our lives but contribute significantly to healthy ageing.

The question this book explores is how we break the negative power of the spells these fantasies cast over our lives after we reach the magical age of 50. They are woven into the fabric of our cultures and have come to represent a truth that shapes our beliefs and behaviours. Instead, I will encourage women to replace them with ones that give them permission and encouragement to live life to the full.

I am a passionate, opinionated expert of life beyond 50, having had to navigate the significant milestones attributed with this exalted status some years ago. These have included physical as well as emotional changes, preparing myself for retirement, applying for a part-time job, dealing with ill health, coming to terms with the loss of loved ones and not to mention the oft-ignored milestone of the M-word.

There was either an absence of inspirational information available to help me navigate these rites of passage associated with ageing or extensive academic rhetoric shrouded in medical and research language. Instead, what I would have benefitted from was honest and plain language backed up by personal experience from women who have gone before and whose words of wisdom would have offered comfort.

My journey of discovery also led me to the realisation that longevity is a relatively new phenomenon. We are all learning to deal with the consequences of an ageing population and creating the rules as we go along. There is yet no blueprint for getting older, which can only be a good thing as we get to write the script. So, instead of lamenting the effects of our ageing bodies, sagging body parts, wrinkles in unusual places and aching joints, we can contribute to finding solutions in navigating this unknown territory.

This book, therefore, aims to do exactly that; share stories based on experiences from women such as myself. I will attempt to debunk the oftentimes condescending as well as the medical language associated with getting older. The stories and experiences of other women offer comfort and inspiration knowing others have gone before and not only survived but in many instances thrived. It is also an invitation to dial down the feelings of guilt for just about everything women are so skilled at nurturing and instead dial up the permission to become a bit more selfish and have fun in the process.

We need to recognise that longevity is a gift we should treasure daily, not squander it by resenting getting older and attempting to resist the inevitable. Instead, celebrate and be grateful for each year of getting older. It is a privilege many people have not been able to enjoy. So, make the most of it.

Throughout this book, I will share my own experiences of life beyond 50 as well as the inspirational stories of many women who have shared their journeys with me. Some stories are heartbreaking whilst others are truly inspirational. I hope the stories will offer inspiration and comfort, realising that others have been in similar situations. It may also serve as a reminder that you are not on your own or the first person to cope with a particular event or set of circumstances associated with getting older.

Although I have written this book mainly with women in mind, there is no reason why you can't pass it on to the man or men in your life. Who knows, it might even go some way in helping them to understand you a bit better. Of course, men have their own experiences and stories to tell as part of the ageing process, but as I have a personal experience of ageing being a woman, my book is therefore written with women in mind.

Setting the Scene

'There comes a point in your life when you need to stop reading other people's books and write your own.'
— Albert Einstein

And that is exactly what I did and this book is the manifestation of following his inspirational advice.

This book sets out to vehemently challenge the deluge of anti-ageing rhetoric that surrounds us on all levels, fuelled by the bombardment from the media. There is a life cycle of all things and we are part of that. I strongly disagree with the denial of age but instead, embrace the ownership of ageing. It is a natural process of life and we start ageing the minute we are born. However, ageing doesn't equate to decline, no matter how hard the media and the beauty industry try to persuade us otherwise.

Why, oh why, does the media, society, medical profession lump us all together in one homogenous group when we reach a certain age? We are unique individuals with our own equally unique personalities and stories who will all experience life as an ageing person in our individual way. We don't discriminate against a group in their 20s in the same way, nor would we lump male and female together as one group.

Yet we do that with the older generation and turn them into an asexual declining body with very little to offer society other than being a burden on the younger generation. As older women, we are only valued by society if we can demonstrate that we are ageing youthfully and actively engaged in pursuing membership of the self-delusional anti-ageing club. The latter being self-perpetuated by the beauty industry to maintain and increase a market for their products.

The only time older people feature in the media and advertising is when they are associated with medical or mobility products such as stairlifts, hearing aids, incontinent pads and any other product you care to mention associated with a declining body. Ironically, have you noticed that these adds often feature, younger and attractive people? It is almost as though we would offend the viewers by portraying people of that particular age. Or perhaps the media is afraid that doing so might shatter the illusion.

What about our very real interests in technology, cars, fashion and again any other product you care to imagine? For many years, I rode a motorbike all year round, a Harley-Davidson to be precise, but I have yet to see an advertisement featuring an older woman as the rider or even as a pillion passenger come to think of it. Normally, that is reserved for gorgeous looking younger women. Also, you do not see older women associated with the latest models in the motor press, even if, like me, you would seriously covet some of the gleaming models.

As far as the media and advertisers are concerned, we cease to function and live a day-to-day life just like any other person under the age of 50. There are some glimmers of hope, however, they are far and few between. As I mentioned in the introduction, there is no guidebook of how we will experience each decade as this homogeneous group. We will all have a very different and yes, I emphasise, unique experience each year we get older.

All isms are socially constructed and if we don't challenge it, we merely reproduce it. In my chapter on 'A Philosophy of Ageing', I talk at length about the socially constructed notion of reality, particularly the experiences of ageing. Ageism is the last socially sanctioned prejudice that goes unchallenged, not to mention robbing society of the vast availability of wealth, experience and accumulated wisdom we have to offer. Here's an interesting point to ponder. Irrespective of any cultural, racial, sexual group you associate with, we all will get older and ultimately be grouped under the heading of seniors, elders, old people, the elderly. Our individuality will miraculously disappear.

We campaign long and hard for recognition of our gender, sexual orientation, identity and race and then when we get old all that goes by the by. It is therefore up to us all, irrespective of the groups we associate with, to challenge the assumptions and discriminations associated with ageing and the diminishment of our experiences and lives lived. By blinding us to the benefits of getting older and putting the fear of God into us of what awaits us as we age, we construct a vision of getting older that is more challenging than it necessarily is or has to be.

At the time of writing, the younger generation is taking the lead and saying enough is enough when it comes to climate change. We need to rethink our treatment of our environment and fast before it is too late. They are showing the way to the older generation and setting the example. By the same token, us as the older generation alive now needs to take responsibility to set the example to generations to come that being over 50, 60, 70, 80, 90 or older is a natural part of life. We also need to shatter the illusion that we are not going to be draining society of resources; that's a myth.

We need to create new rhetoric of anti the anti-ageing brigade. It is our responsibility to be the example, demonstrate how much there is to live for at any age and be the mentors for the next ageing generation. Throughout the book, I will encourage you to be that example and role model. In the first instance, we owe it to ourselves to live the lives we have been blessed with to the full, whatever that means to each one of us.

I will say similar things in different ways throughout the book. This is because we don't always hear or recognise a message when we first encounter it. We also need to hear it in different ways and different contexts before it hits the right note within us. It also depends on our personal circumstances and different people will hear different things at different times.

We are undergoing seismic shifts on all fronts, environmentally, politically and socially. Big questions are uppermost in the news such as how do we get around, should we travel less, what we eat and shouldn't eat in order to stop the ticking clock of destruction to our planet, which is an undeniable and impending reality.

Socially, there is an enormous opportunity for us older women as we don't have to battle outdated ideas and misconceptions of who and what we should do and be. As baby boomers, we are the trailblazers of what it means to age well and express our unique beauty irrespective of age. Our internal beauty isn't eroding or fading. We're old enough to recognise that true beauty never came to us through the eyes of others. It comes from within and shines out.

Despite having lived a number of decades with its myriad of experiences and being drip-fed the doom and gloom of getting older, it has probably taught you to be cautious. Fear creeps upon us as we grow up and age, curtailing our ability to be spontaneous and possibly even impulsive. I will, however, throughout the book apply logic, research and the inspirational stories of other women to address these fears and challenge the perceived doom and gloom that in many instances will probably never materialise.

Thanks to my mother and the genes she passed on to me, I have always been an energetic and positive person, wholeheartedly embracing change and new experiences. However, my 50s were not my best decade and severely challenged my optimistic default position. I nearly succumbed to all the anti-ageing rhetoric for a number of reasons. As with many women before me, I had to embrace changes at a physical, mental as well as emotional level by the time I reached the 50s.

In addition, I had to adapt and manage the changes brought on by the menopause and coping with my husband's health challenges. It was also during my 50s that I lost my beloved brother to terminal cancer, leaving a big hole in my life.

Furthermore, I took early retirement and found it quite difficult adjusting to the experience. However, over the last two years, I have returned to work on a part-time basis, which has given me a new lease on life. I realised that retirement was not necessarily an all or nothing scenario, but that I could tailor work to suit my circumstances. More about that in the chapter 'Half in or All out'. However, since turning 60, I have had a new injection of energy and zest for life and I have labelled my 60s as the swinging 60s!

I realised that we spend so much time living a life that we forget to take time for life itself, enjoying the little things and moments that truly give joy and make life worth living. Furthermore, as we start our adult life, with all its demands, we quickly give up on our dreams and passions. Deep down, I had a longing to pursue my first love of creativity, design and colour and slowly this is creeping back into my life.

Pursuing a career in the creative field was not going to happen. My father expected me to get a 'proper' job with regular hours and income and not as he saw it, the unconventional life of art and design. Since retirement, it has taken me more than two years to finally give myself permission to dare open the padlocked box that contained my unfulfilled dreams and desires. I finally understood the inspirational quote by Maya Angelou, 'Success is liking yourself, liking what you do and liking how you do it.' Often the career successes we strive for are transitory by nature.

My career spanned many years working with people on a 1:1 basis as an executive coach as well as groups of adult learners in an educational setting. The common thread was supporting individuals in their development, recognising and realising their inherent potential. My career has therefore provided me with the privilege of being entrusted with the personal stories of many individuals on their unique journeys.

How we overcome some of the challenges life puts in our path or embrace new opportunities that come knocking on our door will solely depend on our attitude towards them. As with trees, we can choose to bend and flex and therefore survive and grow or become rigid, inflexible and inevitably snap and break in the buffeting winds. This is a fact supported by cognitive behavioural psychology. Our attitude to experiences and the meaning we assign to them will largely determine how we react. To emphasise, we respond to our interpretations of events and not the events themselves.

Many of us would have shared similar experiences during our lifetime. However, I can guarantee that we would all have had our interpretation of these events and therefore responded in a way that reflected our assumptions and views about the world. I will explore the influence and power of our assumptions on our behaviours in later chapters.

No doubt you will raise numerous reasons and excuses why my suggestions for viewing the world differently could not possibly work or is not relevant to you or…fill in the gap with your own excuses. I am, of course, not familiar with your circumstances, so how could I possibly know and understand how difficult it is or how complex your unique situation may be.

However, I am a very tenacious person and I will not let you off the hook that easily. Not without a struggle or a very persuasive argument to keep you doing from what you have always done or be what you have always been. My invitation and challenge will be to encourage you to go off-piste now and then and do things differently, in a different order or different things altogether. You might just surprise yourself with how rewarding this can be.

We will chat, laugh, cry and exchange experiences. I can guarantee that I will be controversial and ignore many of the politically correct norms with which we dutifully collude. Furthermore, I will challenge you to think of life in different ways and from different perspectives. My belief is that there is always more than one way to look at life and the unexpected surprises it puts in our path. As an academic, wherever possible, I will support my assertions by research, some of which I provide in the list of resources at the end of the book.

Just in case you have missed what I said earlier or chosen to ignore it, you will notice a specific thread that weaves its way throughout the book, namely that of attitude. It is not only my experience but also my deep conviction that whatever we encounter in life, our attitude is critical in how we deal with it. Attitude determines the quality of those experiences or prevents us from recognising and embracing their hidden gifts. I'll support this assumption with the many anecdotes from inspirational women as well as men who have challenged the norms and beliefs of getting older.

One of my many passions in life is having stimulating and engaging conversations with interesting people, or as my cockney friend would say; nothing like a good old chinwag. It is probably why my career took the path that it did. Furthermore, I saw my purpose as challenging the boundaries of knowledge and to create a love of learning about self, life and whatever the subject we were exploring. I also see the challenge of the boundaries we create, stifling our personal growth and development whilst at the same time depriving us of many of the joys of life.

This book is therefore an invitation for you to join me in a conversation. As you read, I want you to imagine that I am sitting there with you in your sitting room, study, kitchen, lying in bed, sunning yourself on the beach or wherever you enjoy doing your reading. Each one of us is ageing, but our experiences will be unique to each of us and hopefully, you will find inspiration from the stories of others on your ageing journey.

So, put on the kettle as my mom was fond of saying and let's start chatting...

What Our Cultures Say About Ageing

'Age is an issue of mind over matter. If you don't mind, it doesn't matter.'

–Mark Twain

Ageing is so much more than merely a biological process. It is also associated with deeply rooted beliefs mirroring our cultural norms. Cultural beliefs significantly influence the way we perceive the ageing process in both ourselves and others. Throughout this book, I challenge the anti-ageing rhetoric and instead offer an alternative view that suggests ageing is an unprecedented period of human enrichment and fulfilment.

Our cultural beliefs and expectations of ageing significantly dictate so many interactions with the older generation and the assumptions we harbour of that particular group. A particularly annoying experience I had recently is an example of this.

Following various conversations with NHS111 in order to obtain an emergency prescription for my husband, I had the displeasure of speaking to a condescending young man who clearly perceived me as an older woman with failing capacities. He would have been aware from my husband's details that he was in his mid-70s and therefore made an assumption about my age. He was downright rude, constantly interrupting me and in a patronising manner kept calling me 'my dear' until I interrupted assertively and pointed out that I was not his dear. I further suggested he had the choice to address me as either Mrs Davies or Dr du Toit.

For anyone less confident or assertive, they would have been railroaded. I was so incensed at the experience and the example of being dismissed, questioning my intelligence and mental capacity based on my perceived age. It was interesting when merely five minutes later, I received a call from a GP endeavouring to sort out their incompetence.

On the one end of the continuum, ageing is perceived as undesirable due to the loss of beauty and the possible onset of illness, taking us ever closer to death. Whilst on the other end of the continuum, in some cultures, it is celebrated because of the perceived wisdom age brings and the status and respect that accompanies maturity.

For example, there are significant cultural differences to the attitude of social care of the elderly. Western and Japanese cultures strive to ensure independence for as long as possible. On the other hand, some cultures favour family care for the elderly, India being an example. In contrast to Western cultures, including the U.S.A. and the U.K., the Mediterranean, as well as Eastern cultures such as India, China, Korea and Japan, hold the elderly, especially men, in high regard.

In these cultures, traditional cultural values insist on respect towards older people and the perceived wisdom that accompanies age and experience. In China, in particular, this extends to deference and respect for one's ancestors as well as one's parents.

The regard for ageing in Eastern cultures can trace its roots back to Confucian principles, which insist on respect for one's elders. It is the duty of the younger generation to care for the elderly members of their family. The deference for their elders extends to the wider society and includes people in positions of authority.

In Singapore, they go one step further and parents can sue their children for an allowance and if the adult children fail to comply, they could face a jail sentence of six months.

Not only is respect for one's elders in Eastern cultures perceived as one's duty, but it is also considered the highest virtue. Sadly, Western influence is creeping into their larger cities and communities. However, placing one's parents in an elderly home remains a deeply dishonourable act.

In the West, on the other hand, we have been influenced by a Protestant work ethic, which suggests that if you are no longer able to work, you have lost your value to society. This is reflected in the way the elderly is often viewed in certain societies. Our Western societies, in particular, are also highly mobile, which means the elderly may find themselves a long way from friends and family and a support network.

An interesting question is what happens if you do not have children? It is a particular problem in China with its one-child policy. The care and support of elderly parents is therefore the sole responsibility of the only child. Furthermore, as with a rising life expectancy as experienced in the West, the result is an increase in the ageing population with a smaller group of younger generation having to shoulder the burden of social care.

In some cultures, we find generations living together with the elderly perceived as the head of the family. In India, many live in joint family units with the elderly supported by the younger generation. The elders also play a significant role in the raising of their grandchildren. Their opinion and advice are sought on many different matters and more importantly, valued. Where there are disputes, the final word lies with the parents.

During my years travelling to Austria, I observed the same practice in rural communities. The eldest son would inherit the farm and once he marries, he and his wife would live with his parents. In time, they would take care of the parents and assume the responsibility for the running of the farm.

Alas, the older traditions are changing in many cultures and we all face the global challenge of an ageing population. This puts pressure on the younger generation due to an increased need for social care; a wicked problem without easy answers.

Cultural differences also include how we perceive death. In some Western cultures, death is a taboo subject and we avoid talking about it at all cost. It is something to be feared and when it happens, it evokes a strong emotional reaction to the loss of a loved one. However, cultures such as Eastern and native African-American cultures celebrate the passing of a loved one and the life lived. Death is perceived as part of the natural rhythm of life.

Particularly in Western cultures, ageing is viewed negatively and to be avoided at all cost. The older you get the more invisible you become as far as the younger generation is concerned. The media and fashion industries begin to ignore us unless it becomes a political issue, as we are currently experiencing in the U.K. with the ever-growing crisis in social care.

When reaching her 50s, Margarette was surprised to experience a lack of interest from society and felt no longer valued in terms of childbearing nor being of sexual interest. She also no longer felt valued as a mother as her children grew up, became independent and left home. Finding a valued role in society was a challenge for her. On the other hand, the experience was also liberating. For years she had to deal with family pressures of getting married and once having done so, the pressures to fulfil what society expected of her role as a woman, namely to have children. Now, no one asks of her what she was going to do next and she has found that freeing, leaving her to explore and experiment with interests and activities she has never had the time or space to explore.

The crisis of social care across continents reflects the negativity associated with age and the perceived burden it places on society. Is it any wonder, therefore, that we fear the process of ageing thereby creating self-fulfilling prophecies as we age instead of living life to the full? It will surprise many of you to learn that only about 4% of the population will actually require long term care in a care home. Yet, even scientists have made reference to the so-called problems of ageing.

Given what I've just said in relation to long-term care, why should ageing be seen to be problematic? At 60, I feel much better than I have ever done at a younger age. This includes health, confidence and above all contentment with life. I, therefore, encourage you to change the mantra of inevitable physical and mental decline as we get older and instead, choose to improve with age focusing on joy, creativity and curiosity.

At the time of writing, society is divided into so many lines such as race, religion and immigration not to mention politics and an ugly resurgence of anti-Semitism across Europe. The media fuels these divides with comments that pit the older generation against the younger ones. What most people fail to realise is that a drip-feed of negativity towards ageing is absorbed subconsciously and ultimately producing significant negative beliefs about ageing and what the future may hold for all of us.

These comments suggest the ageing population is bankrupting the National Health Service in the U.K.; enjoying pensions and state benefits paid for by the younger generation who will not be able to enjoy the same level of benefits when they retire; older people take the jobs younger people should have due to higher retirement age.

This polarisation between generations seems to have escaped countries such as Japan. As a culture, they appear to have truly achieved an intergenerational society. Job roles are performed by people anywhere from 20 through to those in their 80s. With life expectancies increasing, we are on the threshold of how we as a society deal with age and ageing and countries like Japan seem to have it nailed.

Society includes multi-age consumers, so why should we therefore not have a multi-age workforce? It is probably also the only way to sustain an ageing population, many of whom want to contribute financially to society, yet find it difficult to do so due to outdated beliefs about ageing and the older generation.

Older people are often portrayed, as a burden society is unable to afford. If we pause and think about it, at many stages throughout our lives we rely on others for support and survival. We would not grow into healthy, productive adults if not for the many years of nurturing and support from our parents and others.

The result is that many older people feel guilty, ashamed and useless. Feeding and accepting this negative story leads to a self-fulfilling prophecy, reducing life expectancy and quality of life. However, there are alternative views supported by research that suggests the health care expenditure is, in fact, insignificant in comparison with the burden on the health care system from other factors such as obesity, alcoholism and the associated diseases with an unhealthy lifestyle often inflicting the young rather than the old.

Let's not forget how many grandparents contribute significantly to society by offering free childcare to their grandchildren. I am aware that there are grandparents on both sides of the argument and no doubt my comments will reflect this. Many of you who have shared your experiences as grandparents with me, reflect the joy in spending time with your grandchildren. However, the other side of the coin is that grandparents should not become a slave to their families. One woman who shared her stories with me suggested it came to a point where she felt she had to get permission from her daughter to go on holiday!

Although being a grandmother is a very rewarding role, you are also a woman in your own right, with experience, skills, dreams, needs and a lot of life that still needs to be lived. You are not simply 'just' a grandmother. A significant number of women who take retirement see it as an opportunity to indulge in new adventures and often, new careers. Unless it is your choice, do not collude with your family into becoming a full-time childminder. Remember, you are being an example to the younger generation that there is much life to be lived throughout life, even and especially after retirement.

Many researchers suggest that the efforts spent on the negative aspects of ageing need to be balanced with research highlighting the positive aspects of getting older. A similar crisis occurred in psychology, which has traditionally focused on the deficits of the human psychological condition. The positive psychology movement has spent its energies and research highlighting the positive aspects of the human condition.

The sense of wellbeing associated with positive psychology does not dismiss that we all face challenges throughout life or the possibility of eventual decline of different aspects of the body. The critical difference is how we approach and deal with these experiences. Throughout, I will challenge the prevailing arguments with current research and of equal importance, the experiences and stories offering alternative points of view.

Beauty and the Hag

'I found out a long time ago it's more fun being the wicked witch than the helpless princess.'

– Tammy Faith

You may have, no doubt, mused over my choice of the book title and possibly even felt offended by older women being referred to as hags. There is a good reason for it. In the first instance, in keeping with my belief in the power of attitude, it is healthy not to take ourselves too seriously.

At the beginning of the writing process, I proposed the reference of hags to a large group of women through an online network and was intrigued by the vehement reaction from a number of them to the chosen name of my book. How dare I call older women hags, even in jest! This stimulated my curiosity and I decided to delve some more into the reason for such an emotive response. In order to do so, I turned to fairy tales to find the answer.

Irrespective of the cultures in which we grew up, fairy tales are awash with innocent damsels in distress, villains, heroes and, of course, wicked stepmothers, witches and hags. Throughout, fairy tales perpetuate the stereotypes of women as either passive, beautiful and young and in need of rescue by the handsome price, of course. Alternatively, they are portrayed as embittered older women embodying evil, ugly and often deformed and to be despised and feared. The women in my survey did not want to be associated with the older, evil women of the fairy tales that had evoked such fear in them as children.

Consider the characters of the fairy tales and the beliefs associated with the various stages as we develop, especially for those of us in the 50+ bracket. We start with the beautiful and innocent young girl who attracts the brave and handsome prince to live happily ever after. Over time, she ages and her physical appeal begins to fade and at some point, she becomes invisible morphing into one of the embittered, ugly hags or witches.

Powerful, older women who stand up for themselves are often depicted as murderers, child-eating witches or hags. On the other hand, the timid, powerless heroine has to be saved from the clutches of the evil, older women by the handsome prince charming. In most fairy tales, these two stereotypes are pitted against one another. The message is that passivity and beauty are rewarded and older, powerful and strong women are often punished by death.

The subconscious message is that women are weak and vulnerable and can only succeed when a man intervenes on her behalf. We can observe the continuation of the theme of powerful women as villains in many cultures. Successful women leaders, whether in business or politics, are often portrayed as cold, heartless and manipulative or worse.

Fairy tales unashamedly instil fear of older women in children. How often do parents use these characters to threaten and cajole children who misbehave? In fact, when you analyse some of the stories we regale to children before bedtime, it is not surprising that they experience nightmares. The wretched witches lure children into their den to be roasted in their ovens, cast evil spells on them or lock them away in towers.

Apart from being blood-curdling gruesome, vilifying older women in fairy tales is particularly scary because the most powerful person in the life of the child is the mother. There appears to be an underlying fear of female power in ancient tales told across different cultures. It was, of course, not all that long ago that the fear of such power resulted in witch-hunts to rid society of their threat, devious and immoral behaviour. The response to the suggested title of my book gave me a glimpse into the power of illogical collective thinking, resulting in the condemnation and persecution of women in the middle ages.

However, in some cultures, older women are revered in stories as they are seen as the ones who keep the family together, pass on traditions and who are wise and knowledgeable in the art of magical remedies to cure all illnesses. In these folklores, older women have the power to judge, punish, reward and heal and therefore assume the centre characters of the stories.

During ancient times, the crones, hags and witches were frequently sages, leaders, midwives and healers within their communities and were revered for their wisdom and knowledge. As history evolved and a patriarchal society took hold, the definitions of the crones (the crowned one), the hag (the holy one) and the witch (the wise one) were distorted.

It, therefore, does not come as a surprise that as older women, we fear the loss of our youthful appearance as the older and wicked women of the fairy tales are often portrayed as gnarled, grotesque and physically frightening. It might very well be that the hags of our stories may have a gift to give us, namely to push back at life, individuals and relationships that have been all-consuming. Have the courage to claim back some of your space and learn to say 'no'.

On the other hand, the stereotype of youthful beauty being the ideal is constantly reinforced and upheld as the holy grail by the media and the beauty industry. I argue that the result is detrimental to the physical as well as mental health of young women. The modern twist to the tale is that although women may assume a more powerful and independent role, they have to remain physically attractive. The media and glossy magazines continue to perpetuate the myth that you have to be beautiful to be successful.

Throughout our history, mankind has always used storytelling as a way to describe and share the history of the tribe therefore ensuring their legacy was protected. It is through stories that we come to understand, learn and know. Stories are a powerful means through which we develop a sense of self.

It is worth remembering that stories may also contain the truth as well as lies and deception. For example, the lies we tell ourselves about how we should feel, behave and be when we get older. If we tell ourselves a story often enough, we will begin to believe it. The stories society and the media tell about ageing is about fear and decline. Yet, there is an alternative story.

Furthermore, we are unaware of how the constant bombardment from the many forms of media permeates our lives to influence our identities and beliefs through the stories they beguile us with. The negative stories of ageing they tell us infiltrate our subconscious minds to shape our expectations and experiences of ageing. Science has proved that the negative stereotypes surrounding the process of ageing are as pervasive as they are inaccurate.

The media portrays an image of older people and how they live based on the lifestyle of the previous generation. Instead, we should identify and celebrate appropriate role models to reflect the current reality of people over 50; the third chapter. Women become much more vivid as they get older. There are so many possibilities if we want to acknowledge and own it. We have more capacity than we give ourselves credit for. I suggest the world is, in fact, opening up to older women and not closing down as we are led to believe.

Older women have the ability to polarise society. One such a woman is Maggie Thatcher, who came to power as the first female prime minister in the U.K. in the late 1970s. Whether you loved her or hated her, she was a powerful woman who made a significant contribution to breaking the glass ceiling and how our perception of powerful, older women has and continues to change and evolve.

Most of us of a certain age would have been brought up with the iconic image of the comic book character *Wonder Woman*. As women, we collude with nurturing the stereotype of women needing to be wonder woman in every aspect of their lives and perpetuating the guilt many working mothers face, juggling all the demands on their time.

I was fascinated to discover that the United Nations as recently as 2016 appointed the 75-year-old heroine as its new honorary ambassador for the empowerment of women and girls. However, the outrage with which the news was greeted was not, I would imagine, the response the UN would have expected. An online petition, arguing that Wonder Woman was not an appropriate choice, attracted more than 1000 signatures.

I quote from the petition, 'a large-breasted, white women of impossible proportions, scantily clad in a shimmery, thigh-baring bodysuit with an American flag motif and knee-high boots – the epitome of a 'pin-up' girl', summed up the mood of the signatories. The general tone was one of anger that the UN could not find a real-life woman able to represent the rights of all women in the fight for their empowerment.

The Amazonian princess was created by the psychologist, William Moulton Marston in 1941 and inspired many of the leaders of the suffragist movement and seen as a feminist icon for many years. In defence of the UN, she was perceived as the first female superhero among an army of male superheroes and her purpose was always to fight for fairness, justice and peace.

The announcement outraged women around the world given the fact that the headlines in the United States reflected the objectification of women and girls. It is seen as alarming that an icon of an over-sexualised image should be perceived as an acceptable representation of women's rights.

There are so many women and girls around the world who continue to suffer not only discrimination but violence and abuse of the worst kind. In many instances, such violence results in death. Where such violence occurs, it often goes unpunished, hence the need for a strong ambassador. The purpose of the role is to raise awareness of these atrocities and act as a conscience to society for the purpose of changing the circumstances of many of these women and girls.

It is therefore difficult to understand what message the UN was trying to send out about the representation of strong women. Given the many credible women able to represent the issues, why would the cartoon of a woman seem to be appropriate in reflecting the importance of the new role? Whether we agree or not, it seems a rather ill-informed choice that was bound to evoke strong feelings and rejection. It confirms the assertions I make in this chapter regarding the power of stories in our lives.

As individuals, we too have stories to tell about our lives and the characters we have and continue to play. Central to storytelling is the concept of interpretation, which suggests that meaning is fluid and contextual and not fixed and universal. It further suggests that our life stories remain open-ended, allowing us to re-author our stories to enrich our lives rather than impose limiting constraints on our experiences. By deepening our understanding of the meaning of our personal stories, we are able to create new stories that better reflect the woman we have and continue to become.

The story of ageing is a powerful example of a meta-narrative, which we all collude with. However, as storytellers, we are powerful in our ability to influence how our stories will turn out. Our identities are imbedded and influenced by the cultures, which we inhabit and interact with and are therefore multi-voiced. However, we do not need to become prisoners to the stories told by our cultures. We are the author of our own stories and can therefore choose to change the plot and the characters.

Research supports the fact that the stories we tell ourselves will come to pass and tests have shown that how we think about getting older in terms of decline or disability will be reflected in the state of our health. This is not to say we should deny experiences of decline in physical strength and some abilities. However, it is vital to separate fact from fiction.

Ageing is not merely a physiological process and the stories we tell ourselves about ageing also have a significant psychological influence on the quality of our lives. I invite you to reflect on the stories you tell yourself. Are they negative and inaccurate or uplifting and life-enhancing? You are in charge of the stories you tell about your life. Choose wisely.

By choosing the title of H.A.G.S. for my book, my aim is to contribute to the rewriting of the ageing story of older women and reinstate them with the wisdom and respect they deserve. Let us take a lesson from the fairy tales and remember that it is the older woman who can work magic for both themselves and others.

The Power of Attitude

'A positive attitude may not solve all your problems, but it will annoy enough people to make it worth the effort.'

– Herm Albright

The A in H.A.G.S. is all about our attitude to life and ageing. As I stated in the introduction, our attitude to life and getting older is central to this book. Attitude is one of the significant factors that will determine the quality of life and its many experiences. Research findings suggest that our general attitude and perception of our ageing hugely influences both physical as well as psychological experiences in later life. It is therefore fitting for me to share my beliefs of attitude with you as it applies to the journey of getting older.

In Europe, we are somewhat reserved towards what we perceive as gushing emotions or a Pollyanna approach to life. I, therefore, support many of my assertions with scientific research to back it up. It's a fact of life that the pawpaw hits the fan occasionally, but what is of importance, as I will constantly remind you, is our attitude towards it.

We have the choice of being down, miserable, unhappy, feeling done by or we can choose to be upbeat, positive and grateful for what we have. Whichever choice we make will become a habit and ultimately a self-fulfilling prophecy. If our thoughts constantly centre on the negative, we contribute to paving the way to physical and emotional ill-health. The converse is true, therefore, choose what will expand and not contract your life and let that become your truth and reality.

We hugely underestimate the power of language, reflecting the values we hold and contributing to our world and its experiences. Sadly, the media significantly influences the attitude of society towards ageing. As older women, it is necessary for us to be aware of the anti-ageing messages and avoid colluding with their rhetoric. The beauty industry constantly bombards us with anti-ageing lotions and potions to help stave off the process of ageing. These messages reinforce the deep-seated cultural aversion to growing older. A small but powerful example I noticed a couple of days ago. The hand cream I am currently using, clearly states in bolder letter 'anti-ageing'. I stopped to reflect what this said about me and my own subconscious beliefs about ageing. We do not label other products in the same way, perhaps except for baby products. Why can't such labels be rephrased as 'care for the older or mature skin', or words to this effect? The media ensures we are made to feel guilty for ageing. We are punished for losing our youthful appearance as ageing is treated as a sin and we have transgressed!

Instead, I feel passionate that we should be celebrating our years and our achievements rather than be ashamed of the decades we have lived and loved. They have all contributed to the women we have become. Instead of being made to feel guilty, we should be encouraged to be grateful for the years we have had to amass our experiences and discovered all those wondrous aspects of what makes us who we are. Instead of shame, we should give thanks to each year we have been on this beautiful planet of ours. It is worth taking the time to count our blessings and to reflect on what we take for granted. As I will remind you throughout this book, the best way to age healthily is to age fully engaged and with gusto.

The positive aspect of attitude is how we as older women choose to view life and the way in which we express and engage with life at a given age. Without recognising it, as women we internalise the cultural fears associated with getting older. Sadly, many women bring about what they fear through their lifestyle and critically, their attitude. Negative self-perceptions and attitudes impact our health, physical functioning and cognitive abilities.

I recall my mother saying when she turned 50, she didn't conform or keep quiet anymore. For her, fifty came with the courage and attitude to express her opinions and concerns and even to say 'no' to requests and demands made by others. After a lifetime of navigating the expectations of her husband, children, parents, friends and society, she had found her voice and the courage to express it. In a conservative, male-dominated culture, this was quite courageous.

It is not only my experience but also my deep conviction that whatever we encounter in life, our attitude is critical in how we deal with it. I am also encouraged by the stories I've gathered for my book and the experiences of other women confirming that there is also much joy, creativity and gifts to be discovered as the years unfold. Many of these women were determined not to be defined by a limiting script imposed by society and its expectations of what life should look like as we get older. These women saw retirement and later life as merely an extension of endless possibilities.

Just one of many examples of women who testify to this is Tricia Cusden, who at the age of 66 when others consider retirement, founded a company called, Look Fabulous Forever, offering a make-up-line and skincare for the over 50s. Having used many of the products, I can highly recommend them based on personal experience. The company has continued to go from strength to strength.

My approach to getting older reflects my philosophy of life in general, namely, that our attitude is the most significant factor that will determine the quality of our experiences. I am delighted to have discovered a significant amount of research that supports this assertion. Ageing with a positive attitude is therefore a recipe for better physical and mental health. Apart from the health benefits, having a positive attitude is also likely to ensure that you have a healthy social life.

As part of the research for this book, I stumbled on an excellent idea to remind us of the positive things that happen in our daily lives. The suggestion is that at the beginning of a new year, you take an empty tin, box or any other container and on a weekly basis, reflect on one good thing that happened that week, write it down and put it in your gratitude box. On New Year's Eve, take out your gratitude box and read about all the good things that happened to you during that year. It is a powerful reminder that more good than bad things come our way.

There is also a very practical reason why we need to pay attention to our attitude in life, particularly as we age. Research proves beyond doubt that a positive attitude about ageing not only prevents future ill health but that it also helps to keep the mind sharp and active. Furthermore, it confirms that a negative attitude is likely to significantly contribute to both physical and cognitive frailty. The findings go on to propose that gratitude has a positive impact on the heart and in general also leads to better sleeping patterns.

A woman I was talking to whilst waiting to join an aquafit class at the swimming pool of my local leisure centre reinforced this very point. In her 70s, she shared how she has to hold on to both rails when coming down the stairs due to arthritis in her knees. Her discomfort was the reason for joining aquafit classes in the first instance. Yet, giggling like a teenager, she shared the fact that the evening before she was boogying the night away! She proudly continued that although her dance routine was not as energetic as in her youth, she certainly held her own. She embodied the advice of science that with the right attitude, we should not allow creaking joints and aches and pains to prevent us from enjoying that which brings us joy.

Gratitude results in higher levels of positive emotions, satisfaction with life, vitality, optimism and lower levels of depression and stress. People who value the good things in their day-to-day lives rather than obsessing about ageing are also more contented with life in general. It is the capacity to be able to savour the everyday experiences from the taste of a comforting cup of tea or coffee, a piece of exquisite cholate, a genuine smile offered by a stranger to the breathtaking and unexpected beauty of a sunset. Such positive emotional outcomes can only lead to better physical health. We do not need wealth to experience blessings. In fact, they may deprive us of the joys of the simplicity of everyday life.

Focusing on all those things in our lives to be grateful for boosts our happiness and our general sense of wellbeing. I was pleasantly surprised to discover research that suggests people in their 50s and 60s are happier than they were in their 30s and 40s. We have left behind the years of pursuing career goals and building a home and security for our families. The time is now to examine our attitude towards ageing as the prejudices and negative scripts we indulge in will determine the quality, or not, of the years ahead.

Furthermore, having an attitude of gratitude not only shifts our mindset, but it also serves as the lens required to find solutions to things we want to change. Being grateful, mean we are also more resourceful and open to new and different ways with which to approach challenges or problems we will no doubt encounter from time to time. We always have the choice to reappraise negative situations or emotions in a positive light.

As like attracts like, it will go a long way in helping us to resonate with like-minded people and draw the kind of experiences and people we want in our lives. It is an immutable law of nature and whether you agree with it or not, it will continue to provide you with the experiences you expect. Grateful people do not deny or ignore the negative aspects of life, but instead, choose to deal with setbacks or challenges from a positive and solution-focused perspective. Sometimes a bad situation is a blessing in disguise.

As with anything new, the most difficult aspect is that of making a start. Begin by keeping a gratitude journal, listing those things and events that you are grateful for on a daily basis. The purpose is not to see how many pages you can fill each day, but instead, it will go a long way in creating a feeling of gratitude as your default position.

Express your appreciation for others by saying thank you through notes, messages, texts or emails. It may be a small gesture, but it will have significant consequences not only to the recipient but also you, the giver. Don't underestimate the power of the gift of a genuine smile to a stranger. It might just turn a bad day into a good day for both of you.

Personally, I took the approach that my 60s were going to be my best decade ever. It was my intention to have a year-long celebration of what I termed to be the 'swinging sixties' and take that belief with me throughout this decade. I am determined to rediscover my unique eccentricity and encourage as many of you as possible through my book to do the same. Vanessa agrees and shared with me her surprise at how much she has been enjoying her sixties, despite or probably due to a life filled with many activities and projects.

The added benefit of gratitude is that it snowballs. It is within our power to train our brains to focus on what is positive rather than the negatives of life. Therefore, appreciation and gratitude are emotions we should cultivate and practice on a daily basis. Just as with any activity we continue to repeat, it will become a habit with a positive outcome. There is always something to be grateful for, so start today by expressing it.

Living a Purposeful Life

'The meaning of life is to give life meaning.'
– Viktor E. Frankl

One problem many of us confront when retiring is the loss of purpose. Most of the challenges of earlier life no longer feature in our lives. This is no insignificant event as our lives are held together largely in webs of meaning. Whatever decisions we make regarding our lives after retirement, research stresses the importance of having a purpose, a reason to get out of bed in the morning. In fact, a reason that will motivate us to jump out of bed.

Instead of seeing retirement as a loss, it is much more positive to see it as moving into a retirement or part-time retirement rather than having to give up work. Seeing retirement as a release from the bonds of employment allows us to indulge in activities we have always wanted to do or start a new career altogether.

There are also the physical benefits of having a purpose. Having a purpose leads to better sleep. A purposeful life leads to fewer strokes and heart attacks, lower risk of dementia, and less risk of disability, to name some of the advantages. People who have purpose are more likely to be active, thus contributing to their overall fitness. Having a purpose also suggests that we are likely to be optimistic.

So, face your fears and insecurities. The self-talk will try and persuade you that 'you are too old to learn new tricks', 'you can't dance', 'your bad back will only get worse', 'you will look stupid'. Fill in the blanks with your own excuses… Face them, feel the fear and try it anyway by starting small, building confidence and momentum. If you're worried that you are too old, remind yourself that the average life span is 80, so there is plenty of time for experimentation and adventures.

Go back to the beginning and be a novice once again, if that's what it takes. You may be surprised at how much fun it is to once again learn or discover something new. A friend of mine, Mary, demonstrates the value of being age blind at 80 and has taken up learning to play the flute, something she always wanted to do when she was young but never had the opportunity or the time. Her husband, also a music lover, sang in the local choir until he was 93.

Take the time to revisit your past. You may find that your reinvention is strongly linked to who you were many aeons ago. Often a reinvention is linked to love or interests of various pursuits when you were small or an adolescent but shelved for 'a proper job'. I've mentioned my own experience with this in a previous chapter, rediscovering my love of colour and creativity. Your forgotten interests may lead to a new career or simply a new interest in life that puts you in the path of a whole new group of people and experiences.

Traditionally, career paths followed a certain trajectory. It meant working until retirement age, often within the same company or profession, with enough health and wealth to enjoy your perceived well-earned rest. However, retirement has become very individual with a host of options available from half-in through to all-out retirement, a new career or business and everything else in between.

Research supports the idea that engagement in meaningful activities whether, paid, unpaid or voluntary not only benefits the physical and mental health of the individual, but society at large in so many ways. Those of us in the third age represent a significant and largely untapped resource to society. It is up to us to take the initiative and help to influence and rephrase ageism in all walks of life.

As with all the major life events we encounter throughout our lives, retirement brings changes and choices with each one of us having to decide the path we want to pursue. Two critical challenges accompany any form of retirement. The first is having extended periods of free time and identifying the activities with which we want to fill that time. The second challenge is coming to terms with the possible loss of purpose and for many, a loss of identity.

In relation to the first challenge, retirement offers an opportunity for reinvention or fine-tuning your life to accommodate and engage with those activities that reflect your unique interests or building on a previous career. Irrespective of how you choose to occupy your time, it is a phase in your life accompanied by liberation from conformity and the freedom to do what you want with your time.

The secret is to decide what will bring you fulfilment and a sense of purpose. This can be scary as we have spent so many years responding to and doing what others expected of us in our job roles. Having the freedom to decide what you want to devote your time to can be paralyzing as well as liberating.

Not sure what to do with the next phase of your life, a friend of mine, Dilys Price (OBE) is one example of the philosophy of reinvention, not to mention the golden thread of this book, namely attitude. In her early 80s, she is the oldest woman solo skydiver in the world. After she retired as a teacher, she established her charity, The Touch Trust, working with children and young people with learning difficulties.

Her tireless devotion to raising funds for charities meant she was one of the winners of the 'Pride of Britain Awards' three years ago. This prestigious award is one of many she has collected since retirement. Dilys is an inspiration to anyone seeking to discover what the next phase of their lives might and could look like. The skies are literally the limit for Dilys!

I also believe that we cling to a career paradigm that no longer serves the individual employees, organisations or society at large. The older generation is slowly but surely overtaking the younger generation in terms of size, i.e. the number of people occupying that particular category. The result is that a model hell-bent on putting those of a certain age to pasture results in the loss of rich experiences and benefits to all concerned. Instead, there are significant benefits to be had from intergenerational organisations and working relationships.

One such example is the experience of my husband. He was a magistrate for 30 or so years, loved it and was recognised as an excellent chair. However, at the age of 70, he was forced to retire. All the experience and knowledge he had gained over those 30 years would have benefitted new magistrates if he remained and mentored the new generation. Instead, his experience was discarded and treated as no longer having any valuable contribution to make towards society.

He is an example of certain things we get to learn in life that only comes with age and experience. Life beyond 50 can and is as meaningful, powerful and rewarding as life before 50. I argue on a number of occasions that life after 50 is actually more rewarding for many reasons.

I made reference to the loss of identity that often accompanies retirement. In my experience, it can be a significant challenge to those whose life has been consumed by their careers. A first step in supporting you to deal with the absence of your career is to understand your relationship with your job before taking the plunge.

The years in a certain role or profession leads us to confuse our identities with our jobs. Career progress may also bring a sense of status, which could be an integral part of our self-image or sense of self-worth. Furthermore, our workplaces offer us a social and cultural community with rituals and a sense of belonging that we miss once we retire, especially if there is no alternative to replace it with.

The most challenging question for any of us to answer is, 'Who are you?' The majority of us would respond with our job roles, describing what we do rather than who we are. We associate our identities with what we do for a living. The second great challenge is to be happy with what you find.

Our identities come about through our interactions with our social environment, culture, family and particularly within the workplace. Hopefully, our roles will provide us with the opportunity to express our values and unique abilities to benefit both our organisations as well as the wider community in which we live. Our identities are what give us a sense of self and subjectivity. Furthermore, our perception of self will be reflected in the stories we tell others about who we are.

Our identity is intimately bound up with the social units we belong to whether that is related to our working environment or our culture. Each of our identities demands attention and opportunities for expression. Depending on the stages of our lives, our different identities and the importance they assume will ebb and flow with a different identity taking the centre stage depending on our circumstances.

However, there are times when our work identities may be in conflict with our personal and social identities. This is particularly so when our work identities assume a disproportionate importance in our lives. The result is that we begin to believe that we are our jobs. The consequences of such a belief are likely to lead to stress and burnout.

When we meet someone for the first time, the predictable question that accompanies the ritual of introductions is always, 'What do you do?' Instead, the question we need to answer preferably before retirement is, 'Who are you?' We are not our professional labels. They may represent a key aspect of who we are, but they are not the total of our identities.

This poses a particular problem when we lose our role identity through redundancy or retirement. Answering the question 'who are you?' then becomes that much more difficult to answer. The secret of successfully managing life-changing events such as redundancy or retirement is to know who we are, which includes a healthy relationship with our careers. In doing so, we will allow other aspects of our identity to be acknowledged and given expression, providing us with support to deal with the loss of any aspect of our identity.

I reiterate that significant changes provide us with the opportunity for new beginnings. In the case of retirement, it is not only about the ending of one phase of our lives and therefore the loss of identity, but it also heralds a new beginning and the expression of other aspects of who we are. It is about building and rebuilding the concepts we have about ourselves.

Retirement offers the opportunity for reflection, celebrating past successes whilst embracing the opportunity to develop other aspects of our personalities. For some, the loss of identity associated with their careers will be akin to that of the grieving process after the loss of a loved one. Constructing a new life with new identities can be psychologically challenging.

As I said, it is important to note that retirement does not necessarily mean complete absence from the world of work. It is about choice and whether we want to include elements of paid work in our lives or making the most of the opportunities to develop and pursue other interests; paid or not. The key with preparation is that we consciously make those decisions without having them imposed on us externally. That places us in the driving seat.

A comforting thought is that identity evolves and changes and develops as we go through life. Our identities are intrinsically associated with our values and this is a good place to start in understanding who we are beyond the world of work. We find expression in those activities and goals that give us a sense of meaning and contentedness.

Many who are living a fulfilling retirement has taken the time to plan and prepare before the big day and even to 'practice' what it might look like, rather than leaving it to chance. Doing so will allow you to make the necessary adjustments, both practical and psychological before you do it for real. So, my advice is to start planning! If you find it daunting and don't know where to start, seek help from a trusted friend, colleague, someone who has already taken the plunge or a professional coach such as myself. However, don't delay.

Many of us dream of a future that is different from our present. My brother too had dreams and experiences he was going to pursue with his partner when he retired. He never got there as aggressive terminal cancer had other ideas long before he retired.

Too often, we give up on our dreams just when we need to push harder or persist with circumstances, careers or relationships when we actually should quit. The result is we end up with an unfulfilled future we didn't really want. So, take the time to reflect on who you are and whom you want to become and be in charge of the inevitable transition. Whatever reinvention looks like to you, a new career, hobby or a new life elsewhere; live a life of purpose and be a H.A.G.S. with attitude by pursuing the whispers of your inner voice.

A Philosophy of Ageing

'Nobody grows old merely by living a number of years. We grow old by deserting our ideals. Years may wrinkle the skin, but to give up enthusiasm wrinkles the soul.'

– Unknown

I remember when I turned 60 and could legitimately get my prescriptions for free (which I am fortunate not having to make use of at the moment) and be eligible for a senior railcard. My husband who had already reached this milestone was thrilled on my behalf. I, on the other hand, found it absolutely hilarious and couldn't stop laughing. The reason being was that I didn't feel like a senior citizen or even being able to imagine what it should feel like.

Once I managed to stop laughing and thought about it some more, I became aware of how powerful a label such as being a 'senior citizen' could be. Labels have the power to infiltrate our beliefs and erode our hitherto view of the world. If we hear it often enough, we will begin to believe that we are the embodiment of whatever the label suggests. On a practical level, philosophy helps us to understand how we collude with such labels and go on to co-construct ourselves to fit the label.

However, before we can determine whether philosophy has any insight to offer with regards to ageing, we first need to define what philosophy is. In essence, I would suggest that philosophy is the quest for wisdom. It is having a particular way of thinking about the world and everything in it. It guides and influences how we make decisions, the assumptions and beliefs we hold about ourselves, others and our place in the world and ultimately, it results in our behaviours.

In my simplistic way of thinking, I would suggest it is about making sense of our world. Philosophy may therefore help us to make sense of the process of ageing, giving us the tools to dispel the myths and erroneous assumptions we may harbour about the process of ageing. It may also go some way to help us embrace with understanding and acceptance of the next phase of life that each one of us will eventually enter.

Some approaches to philosophy are critical by nature, but not to be confused with criticism. Instead, it attempts to unmask assumptions, correct distortions, dispel ignorance, challenge myths and reach understanding and insight. Each one of us will find inspiration from different schools of philosophical thought. As an academic, I have had the privilege of being inspired by a number of philosophers and their ideas during my career. One of these great masters that have had a powerful impact on the way I look at and live my life has been the ideas of François Lyotard, the French philosopher.

Much of Lyotard's writing is about challenging what he perceives to be the grand narratives or ideologies told and protected by institutions and society. Of importance is the perceived oppression these meta or grand-narratives exercise over our lives. His thinking encourages us not only to become aware of these so-called truths that have a powerful and controlling influence over our lives but of equal importance, how we collude with these narratives and give away our personal power without resistance.

The power of these stories is that they create limiting beliefs and by giving them credence, we collude with creating self-fulfilling prophecies. The fundamental nature of philosophy, namely, to question and challenge assumptions in ourselves and others provide us with the tools to question the validity and ultimately our acceptance or rejection of these meta-narratives.

This brings me back to the notion of labels I introduced at the start of this chapter. If you consider the many labels or categories assigned to people beyond 50 and more, they tend to be either patronising or disabling and everything else in between. I mentioned elsewhere in the book that as a group of older people, we are lumped together in an asexual mass of society whether we are male or female. These labels, or in the words of Lyotard, namely meta-narratives, transport with them beliefs that convey a truth that the majority of society does not challenge or question.

Powerful entities such as the media, healthcare providers, political institutes, to name a few, perpetuate and reinforce these truths. Sadly, we of the older generation passively accept them without resistance and not only do we begin to mould our lives around these, but they also rob us of the sense of who we are as individuals. In the words of Kenneth Gergen, he concurs with Lyotard and suggests we collude with them to create self-fulling prophecies. Gergen advocates throughout his writings that constructs of any kind, including those associated with ageing, do not reflect a reality that is out there. Instead, they come about through the collusion of everyone in society, including us as an older population. The result is a socially constructed truth that we all then live by and which dictates our beliefs and behaviours.

And so, self-fulfilling prophecies are created. We are not our labels and it is within our power to create new and different constructs by which to live our lives. I encourage you to read the newsletter, *Positive Ageing*, hosted by Kenneth and Mary Gergen of the Taos Institute, details provided in the resources chapter. The newsletter is also packed with research findings that support many of the claims I put forward in the book.

The Gergens advocate that we need category or label busters willing to disregard these culturally-induced labels and expected behaviours for the myths that they are, thereby becoming role models for everyone that is privileged to age. Each one of us can make a contribution, no matter how small, by beginning the process of exposing these labels for what they are. Begin with mindfulness about the language you use.

How often would you start a sentence with, 'I am too old', 'I am having a senior moment', 'It's too late for me to start something new', 'I can't wear that at my age'. Add your own phrases and become aware of how constraining and powerful these phrases are in dictating your behaviours and your sense of self. We need new, or no labels at all, to capture the reality of how people are ageing and living positively into their 70s, 80s, 90s and beyond and it starts with each one of us.

We are exposed to a barrage of these stories associated with the anti-ageing rhetoric on a daily basis. A search online, a trawl of books on ageing and any glossy magazine you care to name is hell-bent on finding ways to avoid or halt the inevitable journey of ageing. It is almost as though ageing is seen as an illness to be avoided or cured at all cost.

Those of us who have entered this phase of life is seen as a different species; objects associated with decline and in need of rescuing. Again, an example of Lyotard's warnings of meta-narratives, the ageing narrative promoted by the media and society is one of anti-ageing. How could we possibly be anti a natural process of life? We are not anti-youth, so why should anti-ageing be acceptable?

I came across a very interesting research project that was conducted with a group of 100 older citizens. Half of the group was exposed to positive messages about ageing in a number of ways, for example, flashing computer imaging. The results were that this group exhibited a range of psychological and physical improvements not found in the group who were not exposed to these positive images.

Furthermore, they benefited from improved physical function, such as balance. They also expressed a higher level of positive self-perceptions and positive stereotypes of ageing were also strengthened with negative age stereotypes and negative self-perceptions of ageing weakened. This supports my passion for us not to collude with the outdated views of ageing found in daily conversation within society and reinforced by the media and other institutions.

Age in itself is not a cause but merely a number that indicates how much time has elapsed since birth. It is, therefore, the truth and power we associate with the numbers that lead to the stories we tell ourselves and our perception of how we should be, feel, look and so forth. Resisting the natural process of ageing also results in closing the door on wisdom, creativity, sense of adventure, freedom from the career grind and the expression of our own unique identities.

Philosophy, therefore, provides us with the courage to question the ageing or anti-ageing story and the perceived inevitability that age leads to physical decline, ill health and a reduction in mental capacity. Should some or all of these aspects of ageing occur, there is no reason why it should lead to a decline in the quality of life or a life worth living.

As I mentioned above, the practical aspects of philosophy and the works of great thinkers provide us with the tools to become aware of how we conspire with these stories or meta-narratives as suggested by Lyotard. So, if philosophy is about challenging our assumptions and dispelling ignorance it is worth drawing inspiration from in order to help us understand and question the stories we, and society, tell ourselves with regards to ageing.

Philosophy also helps us to face our mortality. More importantly, it can provide us with a philosophy of life to make the most of the time we have between birth and death. The quality of our stories reflects the quality of the lives we will inevitably lead at any age. What are the stories you live your life by and more importantly, what is the influence they exercise over your behaviours, attitudes and just living in general?

By the time we reach retirement age, we've seen and experienced much in life. These experiences might have left us jaded, disillusioned or even cynical about life and human nature. We have also spent a lifetime chasing the illusory idea of predictability for the purpose of helping us to feel in control of our lives. Much of our working careers have been spent developing strategies, goals and the plans to help us achieve the holy grail of certainty. We believe in the power of logic and analysis with little room for ambiguity.

Yet, occasionally we get a fleeting glimpse of what we may call luck. I also call it the magic of life. Otherwise known as serendipity. As much as science worships at the altar of logic and reason, many of its discoveries can be attributed to serendipity. The history of science is peppered with such happenstance events; the discovery of penicillin, the microwave, the reliable post-it note and if like me you are a lover of champagne, one of the finest results of serendipity!

If we take time to reflect on our lives, we may begin to see how people, places and events appeared as if by chance. These lucky events may seem rare. However, psychology confirms that we make our luck and can create an environment which welcomes lady luck to call more often.

The number one rule is to break out of routine, which is the enemy of serendipity. Cultivate a mindset that is open to unexpected surprises. Stop sleepwalking through life and consciously embrace unfamiliar situations, engage with equally unfamiliar people and ideas. Luck happens to people who not only go looking for it but also expect to find it. As David Stewart, founder of the AGEIST advocates, order off the menu. In other words, do and try different things and be adventures in doing so.

Think lucky and learn to look at situations differently through positive expectations. Perception is key and will go a long way in creating self-fulfilling prophecies. We get what we expect, remember? Rekindle an interest in undirected play and experimentation, which is squeezed out of us as we grow up. Life is serious with no room for play, we are told. Occasionally listen to and follow your intuition and you will be surprised at what you might find.

Retirement, semi-retirement or a change of direction is that perfect time to cultivate more serendipity. We have the opportunity to create more calm in our lives, letting go of stress and anxiety that prevents us from hearing the quiet knock of serendipity. We can slow down and embrace a more flexible approach to life, gaining a healthier perspective as to what is and isn't important. We are more open to what is in front of us when we are relaxed.

Now is the time to take risks by doing things differently and changing old habits. Listen to the little voice and act on those impulses. What is the worst thing that can happen? Serendipity smiles on those with a more relaxed approach to life. Let go of anxiety or at least put it in perspective as it gives us tunnel vision.

There is some truth in the belief that older people are less flexible. As we get older, we become more crystallised in our thinking and lose the openness and curiosity to life and others we had in our youth. However, it doesn't need to be so. We have the freedom to change our attitude and make different choices.

There are no rigid rules of how we should behave or think as we get older. It is up to us to break the rules and create new ones. It is also perfectly acceptable to be playful and have fun even when you are older. Those of you with grandchildren have a good excuse for indulging in playful activities. Those like me who do not have children, give yourself permission to have fun and do not stress about what others may think. Their thoughts are their problem.

Youthfulness is not exclusively reserved for youth. It is a state of mind available to us all no matter what age we are. It is the capacity to appreciate life and all the gifts it brings and the ability to be surprised with unexpected joys and delights. Youthfulness allows us to remain curious and open to new experiences. In fact, I would suggest that it is only as we get older with life experiences under our belts that we can appreciate and engage with youthfulness.

We are better equipped to let go of unnecessary anxieties about life and ourselves and just be. So, cultivate fearlessness and willingness to try and experiment with something new or different. Instead of thinking of all the things that could go wrong, another symptom of getting older, be bold and give it a try.

Ultimately, I believe it is vital to have a philosophy for living to support us in enjoying a better life as we get older. A practical philosophy has the ability to support us both emotionally as well as psychologically, significantly influencing our wellbeing both mentally as well as physically. I remind you once again that our attitude massively dictates our wellbeing at every level.

A further reminder, it is our thoughts that determine our emotions that eventually materialise in physiological reactions in our bodies. If these thoughts are constantly of a negative nature, they may result in physical and mental problems. It is, therefore, vital for us to be aware of our assumptions towards ageing and guard against colluding with the bombardment of negative images and beliefs about the ageing process.

Embrace the Inevitable

'Beautiful young people are accidents of nature, but beautiful older people are works of art…'

– Eleanor Roosevelt

Let's face it, the only creature that looks cute and cuddly with sagging and wrinkling skin is a Shar Pei. Unfortunately, not for the rest of us, especially if you are a woman conscious of your appearance.

One of my husband's granddaughters offered me the quintessential wisdom of the child when she recently made reference to my 'creases'. Needless to say, she was referring to my increasingly visible wrinkles. However, it made me laugh and I decided that a much more positive approach in viewing my wrinkles was to think of them as creases instead.

I was reminded of the fact that it has been some time since I received a compliment of any description related to my appearance. It has been known for me to be stopped in the street by strangers and being complimented on an exceptional derrière. I hasten to add that it was a long time ago.

In any event, it will no doubt fly in the face of politically correct behaviour in contemporary society. Fascinating how such correct behaviour may not be quite so offensive as you get older! Remember the wolf whistle of days gone by. Sadly, not really…

It is an inevitable, unavoidable, scientific fact that as we age everything; jowls, neck, underarms, décolleté, not to mention the derrière, heads south. As with anything unavoidable, we have a choice in how we respond. But why does it happen and is there anything we can do to slow down the process?

As is to be expected our heredity, body type and lifestyle will all add to the inevitable. There is also the marching of time and the annoying fact of gravity that works against us. Eventually, what used to be firm and bouncy becomes loose, floppy and droopy.

When we age, fat naturally atrophies and the skin becomes loose which gives the important parts of the body a saggy look. As is to be expected, oestrogen or estrogen, or the lack of it, once again rears its ugly head and is the main contributor when it comes to influencing our ageing bodies.

After menopause, our oestrogen levels begin to fall and in relation to the breasts, various glands and milk ducts go into retirement and begin to shrink. To add insult to injury, the tissue that makes breasts firm also begins to shrivel and is replaced by fat, which is heavier and, of course, unable to withstand gravity.

A further contributing factor to looser looking skin is due to our old enemy, cellulite. We also tend to lose muscle mass as we age, making its contribution to the shape of our bodies.

By the time you get this far, you are no doubt in a state of depression and reaching for the biscuit tin! Fear not, there are some things within our control that we can do to slow down the inevitable force of gravity. This is different from trying to deny or escape it.

In the first instance, thanks to modern technology, there are numerous ranges of underwear that will comfortably support sagging body parts. It is therefore worth the effort to visit a reputable underwear store or boutique for professional help and fitting. I stress the word comfortable, unlike memories I have of my mother's generation who had to contort themselves into a rubber garment that any S&M mistress would have been proud of!

By now, you know the mantra and would also expect me to make reference to the H in H.A.G.S. and once again stress that eating healthily and maintaining a steady weight is top of the list. The next obvious thing is the G, namely, get up and go as in exercise. However, there is no need to rush to an expensive gym and pay for a membership you are highly unlikely to maintain. Nor is it necessary to pound the pavements jogging yourself into a heart attack or further aggravating arthritis in your knees.

The bottom line, if you will excuse the pun, is to put on your walking shoes and go for a good old-fashioned walk that includes going uphill. Walking has the added benefit of getting you out into the fresh air bringing with it further health benefits. In addition, wherever possible climb the stairs rather than take the lift. So, as the song by Nancy Sinatra goes, *boots, let's start walking!*

Yes, you've got it, a further reminder is the importance of A in H.A.G.S.; attitude is key. The inevitable ebb and flow of life are marked by a number of stages with the preceding one giving way to the next. Each one of life's stages brings with it its own gift and it is for us to both recognise and treasure these gifts.

According to the beauty industry, there is a lot we can do to make ourselves look younger. In fact, I would suggest, the industry insists that we all need to mindlessly pursue this as the ultimate goal. However, the only way to feel younger is to embrace the fact that every one of us is getting older, irrespective of our age. Accept this and celebrate the beauty that comes with each age.

However, looking after ourselves and making the most of our good points is in my opinion a must for many reasons, self-confidence being at the top of the list. Alas, so many women collude with the anti-ageing rhetoric and give up on themselves and live up to the expectation of society to become invisible. We do so by giving up on our appearance, starting with makeup. For some reason, we believe that when we reach a certain age, makeup is no longer acceptable for us. I have yet to find the reason why makeup should only be relevant to young youthful faces.

So many women have shared with me the disappearance of their confidence as they have got older. Makeup is top of the list in my opinion to make us feel good about ourselves and thereby going a long way in restoring our confidence. We don't put on makeup to please others, but instead, we do so to feel good about ourselves. In fact, the routine of doing so communicates a strong message to ourselves that we matter as a woman. It also gives us the power to challenge the invisibility of older women instead of colluding with it. It says look at me, I matter!

As Tricia from Looking Fabulous Forever so eloquently puts, 'Makeup is all about confidence and self-esteem rather than youth'. We owe it to ourselves to make the most of our good points and give our confidence a boost. As I've pointed out on a number of occasions, we also owe it to the younger generation to show that beauty exists at all ages and that good grooming is also a necessary part of getting older. What message do we send out to the younger generation if we stop looking after ourselves and create the self-fulfilling prophecy of the invisible older women? I hope I am inspiring you to rethink your appearance and to take responsibility for making the most of your appearance and step into the world with confidence.

In fact, I argue that makeup is far more relevant to us as we get older than when we are young with fresh faces and glowing skins. Further inspiration from Tricia says it is completely meaningless to claim that 'less is more' when it comes to makeup. As we age, we need colour to support our ageing skins provided by the right makeup and skincare and applied in a way that suits the individual. Furthermore, making the most of our good points is certainly not synonymous with the anti-ageing rhetoric that suggests we can or should make ageing go away.

If we stop and think about it, we learn about ageing as we do with many other things in life through observation. We have watched our family members, parents and grandparents, age over the years. These observations can be powerful, whether they are positive or negative. It is also important to recognise that our lives are so different from those of our parents and grandparents. It is different on both a physical as well as a mental level.

Science has come a long way to keep us healthier for longer and our attitudes have also changed significantly over the years. A 60-year-old 50 years ago would have looked vastly different from a 60-year-old today and our attitude would equally be vastly different. A 60-year-old woman today would expect to live a long and healthy life for at least 20 to 30 years more.

Let us, therefore, set the example for society and our peers of the benefits associated with the later stages of life thereby increasing our sense of well-being and highlight our contributions to society. For example, the older generation becomes important volunteers and mentors to the younger generation. It is also the time when it all comes together and we are able to enjoy the fruits of our long labour throughout life.

Age is marked by a lengthy accumulation of knowledge and experience out of which hopefully wisdom may grow. Some cultures recognise the value and benefit the older generation has to offer society. Alas in other societies, especially the West, the older generation is often discarded and forgotten.

It is the time when we decide what it was all about. Taking the time to reflect on what the purpose of our lives was and the legacy we want to leave behind will help us to make the most of the final stage of our lives.

It is worth reminding ourselves that being young was not as idyllic as we remember, nor is growing old as wretched as the stereotypes would have us believe. If we feel good about how we look and how we feel, we'll be much more open to new experiences, people and opportunities.

If like me you are childless or your children are far away, it is important to make contingency plans for any possible future needs. Planning doesn't necessarily mean a fixed path of action. You can change your mind at any stage whether it is by choice or necessity. Make a list of some of the eventualities that are worth planning for. As an example, I will research the help that is available to support me for as long as I possibly can to remain in my own home.

If that is not possible long term, I will draw up a shortlist of homes that I would feel comfortable living in after taking the time to visit and interview the staff to determine whether it is somewhere I could end my days. Of course, places change and I may very well discover somewhere more suitable, should that day arrive. That is absolutely fine. What is important is the preparation and getting answers and solutions for any questions or fears you may have about future scenarios.

I would also suggest you provide a file with your wishes to someone who will be able to help you follow through on these decisions, should that be necessary. It is far from being depressive and anticipating worst-case scenario. Instead, it gives you peace of mind and frees you up to get on with life and the many experiences that await you until such time when, and if, your circumstances may change. As I have suggested from the outset of the book, don't be the ostrich and stick your head in the sand, but instead plan ahead. That way you are in control and not merely reacting to the wishes and whims of others.

I challenge you to reflect on the idea of embracing whatever age you are and to be fearless after 50 as fear will stop you from pursuing your dreams and keep you a prisoner in the grey zone of conformity.

Half in or All Out?

'Worrying is carrying tomorrow's load with today's strength – carrying two days at once. It is moving into tomorrow ahead of time. Worrying does not empty tomorrow of its sorry; it empties today of its strength.'

– Corrie ten Boom

The pervading rhetoric in relation to retirement is all about the absence of something. It also suggests that the retiree has stopped doing what used to define them. However, retirement doesn't define who we are as it is merely a description of our social status. A job or career provides us with such labels, which helps others to determine whether we are worthy of talking to.

In a previous chapter, I talked at length about the power of stories and how the stories we tell ourselves about our status and identity determines our behaviours and the beliefs we hold about ourselves. Identities are the characteristics we adopt in the various stories we are involved in throughout our lives.

The social identity our careers afford us reflects our membership of a profession or organisation. However, the more meaningful identity for us to take into retirement is that which makes us different and unique from others. At this stage of our lives, we have the freedom to reconsider and define our own identities.

Our stories help us to make sense of our lives and experiences by weaving them together in a coherent whole. Ultimately, we are the authors of our stories, both past and future and we decide the characters or identities we want to play. Our lives don't come to an end just because our career stories do. It is up to us to create a new story as well as a new character for ourselves.

Not only do we tell our own stories, but they are often inextricably linked and intertwined with the stories of others, such as our organisations or professions. Retirement gives us the opportunity to learn new skills and open doors to new experiences and therefore new identities. There is nothing more boring for the listener than someone who keeps repeating their stories which they relate to their career before retirement.

People who cling on to their professional identities are confusing what they did for a living with who they are as a person. Their stories are normally filled with nostalgia and caught in a time warp. In this case, the narrator adopts a victim identity as it robs them of the ownership to write a new story or stories that will enchant and entertain others and also stories of the moment and not about the 'good old days when they were…whatever their title or profession might have been.

The benefit of our histories and past identities is that they can open up possibilities for us to a future identity and a new story, providing a bridge into a new future. This will only be possible if we are willing to cross the bridge into such a future with the past becoming more distant the further we venture into the new one. The future is open and unwritten until we decide to construct a new reality. It is worth remembering that retirement is merely another process of life and not an event. We will continue to evolve and adapt as we have through many other processes we encountered during our lives.

I remind you of the discussions in the chapter on philosophy and the fact that reality is not independent of us, but only manifests if we choose to take action and interact with a particular reality. This means leaving the identity of the victim behind. For some being the victim is preferred over the opportunity to take responsibility and create a new but unknown reality. Retirement is an individualised and personal journey and it is entirely up to the individual what the next phase of life will look like and the activities to be included.

Furthermore, age does not determine the closeness of decline and ultimate death. The possibility of a long life stretches out before us. Therefore, more reason to create a new present and a future offering and embrace a new identity that is waiting to be realised. Age, just as with our gender, race, disabilities are only limits if we allow them to become so.

A good example of a woman who wholeheartedly embraced a new identity in her fifties was Margarette, who left a career of 30 years as a commercial lawyer working in the oil and gas industry. She went back to university and embarked on a master's degree in coaching. She describes it as the most liberating decision of her life. Having faced many years of discrimination in a male-dominated industry and profession left her battle-weary and disillusioned. The decision to pursue a completely different career has changed many aspects of her life and sense of identity.

She reflects on the influence an organisation and profession can have on one's behaviour and sense of self. Having had to compete in a very male-dominated and competitive environment as a commercial lawyer, her sense of self was very strongly defined by her work role. Because of the contentious nature of the work, she felt she adopted an over-confident, forceful set of behaviours and identified herself as a competitive person. This was reinforced by feedback from others and the behaviours that were rewarded in her professional environment.

She now moulds her work to fit her sense of self and is no longer defined by her profession. It also came as a surprise to her that now in her 50s others no longer have an expectation of her to be pursuing anything and rather to start slowing down, although she feels respected for her wealth of experience. However, she has surprised everyone and possibly even herself, by going back to university and completing a master's degree in coaching. Margarette is a good example of someone who although pursued a totally new career, found ways to integrate and benefit from the experience of a previous career spanning 30 years.

Now Margarette has entered a new phase of her life. She finds it liberating not having the same pressure to live up to other people's expectations of her. She sees this phase in her life now as the time for learning through reflection. In one way, according to the calendar, time seems to be rushing by her, but on the other hand, she perceives time to be expanding and to accommodate her new interests. For her, it is a time for rediscovering what she is interested in and becoming reacquainted with who she is.

If we allow society and their anti-ageing stories to rob us of our power, we become objects to be pitied or resented as we need caring and deprive society of resources, which could be made available elsewhere. We are then seen as someone that merely passes the time until death, despite the fact that we may be engaged in and with various activities.

Having happily decided to reduce my working days, temptation recently had me firmly in its grip. It tapped into my human nature to feel wanted and seduced me with the illusion of my own importance. Luckily common sense prevailed in the end.

And the temptation...? Forfeiting my peaceful existence to once again pursue a full-time career opportunity. At first, I was wooed by the flattery of being seen as the expert they needed, not to mention a handsome salary. I fantasised about what I would be able to do with the extra money until the reality hit home that the financial benefits would come with a high volume of time commitments and personal sacrifices.

I visualised a set of scales with on the one side the extra income and professional status and on the other the freedom and control of my workload that I have enjoyed over the last five years. An image of basking in the sun on the balcony of our house in the South of France, enjoying a long leisurely lunch with my husband and walking in the mountains with our Cocker Spaniel came to mind. On the other hand, if I accepted, I would once again be locked in front of a computer screen working on the next research paper. I realised there was no contest.

No doubt those of you in employment would probably struggle to understand my dilemma. However, I made the decision five years ago to step off the treadmill and take semi-retirement, working for myself and selecting to get involved in work that interests me and doing so at my own pace.

Why would I go back to the stress of churning out journal articles, trying to please egotistical reviewers who take sadistic pleasure in their power to reject one's hard work just because they can? Then there are the endless and pointless meetings, being frustrated with the higher education system and single-handedly trying to bring about positive change.

Instead, I now have the freedom to choose what I want to get involved with and the people I want to work with. I make the choice as to what I write, this book being a great example, and where and when it is published. Above all, I have the time to devote to my clients and the intrinsic rewards it brings.

It was a valuable lesson in reminding me of my priorities in life. I would often work with my clients to support them in establishing what their priorities were and the boundaries they needed to create in order to protect those priorities. I, therefore, had to do some self-coaching to answer the very same questions for myself. Priorities naturally emerge once we are clear about what our values are versus the values we allow others to impose on us.

I was fully aware of the price it would exact on my health, should I succumb to the temptation. One of the reasons I took a step back some years ago was due to severe repetitive strain injury, the result of years being hunched over computers. Anyone suffering from the same would know the pain you are in during every waking hour. I learnt to live with it until the level of pain forced me to choose a different lifestyle. Better health, therefore, became a top priority for me rather than a high income.

I also had more time to enjoy what I love doing most, namely working as a coach and the privilege of spending time with fascinating people. My husband and I have had the time to indulge in travelling, enjoying walks in the countryside and making precious memories with family and friends. Did I miss the salary? Not at all. I have lived a different lifestyle with different needs and the rewards were worth every minute of giving up the high salary. It is true that we adjust our lifestyles according to our income.

In celebration of my decision, Scampy, my elderly, Spaniel and I went for a long walk on the golden beaches opposite my house, enjoying blue skies and mild weather. I would not have had the memories of this walk if I were yet again a slave to a salary. It affirmed that I had made the right choice.

Similarly, Margo made the decision to take early retirement. She reflected on how easy it was to let go of a job that she loved and was passionate about. If anyone had told her just how easy it would be, she wouldn't have believed it. Now, together with her husband, they are renovating a house abroad and she further reflects on how much joy she is getting from the manual and physical labour required to carry out the renovations. Given everything I mention throughout the book in terms of health and looking after ourselves, I have no doubt that Margo and her husband are physically, mentally and emotionally much more healthy as a result of the change they've made.

I will now put forward a counter-argument. There is no law to suggest that because you are of a certain age you have to retire. There is also no law that suggests once you've retired you can't go back to the same line of work or start a new career either. However, there is a pervasive assumption both among the older generation as well as society at large that retirement is synonymous with disengagement and non-participation. Not true.

Unfortunately, ageism and out-dated social structures are real barriers to those who want to continue to participate in the workplace. As an academic in the U.K., I am fortunate that ageism is not perceived as a barrier to those who want to contribute to education and research. In fact, the opposite as one has rich experience and knowledge to contribute to the profession.

There is a myth we all subscribe to that says career or professional reinvention is for the young only. However, a successful reinvention is down to the individual and their attitude. There is no one out there who will give us opportunities; we have to create them. Given the longevity and improved physical and mental health we now enjoy in older age, many choose to continue with their careers or view the traditional retirement age as an opportunity to do something new and fulfil long-held ambitions and dreams.

Continuing with work may therefore take on many shapes and sizes from a new career, starting a business or volunteering time to personal causes. Work in whichever form offers many non-financial benefits such as self-esteem, purpose, social engagement and providing a structure to the day or week. Throughout the book, I mention a number of women who have done just that.

Life sometimes throws a pileup of challenges our way such as health problems, job losses, loss of a loved one and, of course, retirement. These experiences may very well facilitate opportunities for reinvention and change. They also take away aspects of our identity, which means we can never be the same people again. That in itself will bring new opportunities.

However, we have to choose and own these changes whether they were voluntary or imposed. When we lose something or someone that has been a substantial part of our lives, it is difficult to imagine a new future without them. Everything we know is related to our past with the future scary and unknown.

So, where do we start? It doesn't have to be a burning ambition. You may very well not have a clue what you want to do and whom you want to be. Sometimes the best way is to experiment with a number of things before you settle on a path that feels right. Start small and let it build. On the other hand, an unexpected opportunity might pass by and if it feels right, grab it. It doesn't have to be forever. Think of it as an adventure of discovery and one thing may lead to another.

Vanessa is an excellent example of a woman who decided to pursue her dreams in her 50s. She started two businesses and went back to university on a part-time basis to complete a master's degree, which she always wanted to do. Apart from the joy she gets from spending time with her children and grandchildren, she runs a successful business and dictates the pace and commitment she is prepared to put into it.

What is unavoidable is that you have to take some action, no matter how small. That's how snowballs are formed. It starts with one snowflake blown along by the wind, gathering momentum, collecting other snowflakes on the way to eventually result in an unstoppable, enormous snowball.

Fellowship and Solitude

'Being alone has a power that very few people can handle.'
— The Minds Journal

We all know intuitively the value of friendship and social connections and why we need the closeness and intimacy of genuine relationships. I'll explore the value of both solitude and connection with others in this chapter. In the first instance, I want to put forward the argument that being a loner is nothing to be ashamed of, nor a disease to be cured.

Let us pause for a minute to define what we mean by friendship. Sometimes it helps to define what something is by deciding what it is not. And what friendship is not is hundreds of online connections on Facebook or any other social media platform. Although virtual friendships can grow close and the use of Skype and FaceTime allows us to stay in touch with people even though we may be thousands of miles apart. I have been grateful for both of these allowing me to stay in touch with my family over the years.

It is to be expected that friendship will mean different things to different people. It may simply be having someone to meet up for a chat and a cuppa or a glass of wine shared companionship or developing deep and close bonds. Apart from the expectations associated with friendship such as attachment, affection, loyalty, mutual respect and goodwill, true friendship is a relationship that is able to survive the test of time and above all remain unconditional.

Whatever our expectations and definitions of friendship may be, a healthy relationship is rarely one-sided and requires two individuals to make the effort to sustain and build on the relationship. It is the willingness to be there for someone else when the chips are down. It also means making the effort to commit time to the relationship. As with anything worthwhile in life, it takes effort and the commitment to invest time to an endeavour before we can begin to enjoy the benefits.

There are a number of ways in which we can develop new friendships with the obvious being through shared activities. Life events also play a key role in creating long-lasting friendships during our lifetime. Many relationships are forged when we enter school for the first time, the shared experiences of parenting, entering the world of work, to name only a few.

Being involved in some type of group interaction, whether through physical activity such as exercise or one with a more social intention, such as learning a new skill, is fundamental to creating and maintaining a positive experience of ageing. It is not the activity or the purpose of the groups that is important, but instead the support we get from being involved in a group. As social creatures, it is the sense of belonging we get from a group that provides us with psychological benefits. When we talk with people and share our stories, life becomes filled with interest, intrigue, and wonder. I offer a reminder again of the S in H.A.G.S., namely the need for social interaction and connection.

Another significant life event is that of retirement and, in fact, it offers the perfect opportunity to meet new people and develop new friendships. If like me you have spent a big proportion of your life engrossed in your career, travelling and moving around, retirement or semi-retirement allows one the time and space to nurture and develop friendships.

It can also be a challenge, though. Retirement reduces the natural pool of colleagues and business associates that are often the source of our social network. The good thing is there are a lot of other people out there sharing the same life event. In another chapter, I discuss the need to prepare for retirement, including the health and emotional benefits of staying connected with others, particularly as we get older and relinquish some of the social connections we had during our careers.

I reiterate, successfully creating a new circle of friends or adding to our existing social group is dependent on the effort we put into doing so. An inspirational woman who decided to do just that was Helen King who founded a group that have mushroomed and spread throughout the U.K., namely togetherfriends.com. Helen and her efforts to provide a platform for women to connect and forge new friendships have also grown into a successful business. She is a further example of what we can achieve if we put our minds to it and not accepting that age is a barrier. Helen's story is not only encouraging, but her network will also give you the opportunity to meet new people who share your interests. I can vouch for it as it gave me access to a whole new group of likeminded women.

The one significant relationship I had the privilege of enjoying for many years was the one with my gay brother. His love and friendship taught me the meaning of unconditional love. He was my confidante, best friend and sounding board. We shared so much laughter, tears, loss and the pain of separation. Yet, I would not have changed anything as it gave me the true gift of friendship. Alas, he died far too young from terminal cancer, but I have so many wonderful memories I can wrap around me like a cosy blanket when I feel lonely or in need of the unconditional support he so lovingly offered.

Don't forget pets when thinking about unconditional love. I am a huge animal lover and have had the joy of growing up with many animals from dogs to snakes and everything in between. I am sure fellow pet lovers reading this book will agree that pets are abundant in offering continuous unconditional love and unwavering companionship.

If you find yourself living on your own and in need of additional companionship, you will not go wrong with adopting a furry friend. Just make sure it is the right pet for your circumstances and preferences. No point in adopting a greyhound or other animal that needs excessive exercise if you are not fit and enjoy hiking outdoors in all weathers.

I am a firm believer that the most important relationship in our lives is the relationship we have with ourselves. The quality of all other relationships will flow and be influenced by the one we have with ourselves. Take time, therefore, to be with yourself and get to know who you are and offer the unconditional love and acceptance we are willing to offer others. You deserve it as much as they do.

There is significant pressure on us to demonstrate that we are team players in the world of work and it has become a key factor in career success over recent years. Granted so much has been written about the value of teams and the overall argument put forward is that a team can be so much more successful and achieve a great deal more than the sum total of the individual skills. The obsession with teams and groups means that not to prefer to be a team player is an anathema. It also places a significant break on your career.

It is true that as humans, we are social creatures and we tend to seek out the company of others. However, there are also those of us who at times prefer our own company without constantly having to be surrounded by others. I for one cherish my times on my own for reflection, planning, creating or being out in nature and enjoying the natural world. On the other hand, I also love the company of stimulating conversation with the right people.

It is much more rewarding being on your own than spending time with energy vampires that suck the will to live out of you. The response of society at all levels to people seen as isolated is to try and reform the 'lonely' person. The loner is pitied and everything is done to try and fix the situation whether the loner wants it or not.

Different people have different levels of aloneness they can tolerate. The benefit of either complete retirement or reduced working commitments means that you have the luxury of choosing selective loneliness without having to justify it to either team obsessed organisations or the wider society. Finally, you can select solitude without justification or guilt.

Being alone is another aspect of ageing that is a victim of stereotypes and ageist assumptions. An older person on their own is more likely to be the subject of sympathy than a young person. They are very likely to be perceived as being lonely and that may very well be the case. However, it is important to recognise that people of all ages can be lonely and it is not something that merely happens to the elderly. Furthermore, many older people have good social relations and living alone does not necessarily mean they are lonely.

The benefit of having more time to yourself is that you can dictate the pace at which you want to do things. It is within your power to choose to do or not do certain things without having to weigh up the pros and cons of not including someone else. This may seem the act of a selfish person. However, for the loners among you, now is the time to enjoy the luxury of that coffee or shopping trip on your own and at your own pace when you choose. I enjoy meandering around the shops, sip a coffee in my favourite coffee shop and watch the world go by, attend a concert or art gallery, go for a walk as much on my own as with someone who shares my interests.

However, solitude may be a challenging adjustment for those who have been surrounded by others most of their lives and who prefer being in the company of others. Not being prepared for it will be a shock to many retirees. There are so many benefits to solitude, but as with many activities or art forms, it takes practice if it doesn't come naturally to you.

Our careers provide us with structure and social life, which when we retire, may disappear. To some this may be a longed-for blessing, indulging in the many activities they have looked forward to pursuing. On the other hand, if you haven't created a social life beyond your career to suit your personal preferences, it may mean you are deprived of most of the social contact you enjoyed as a result of your career.

Many people think that planning for retirement means financial aspects only. Although critical, it is no guarantee of a successful and contented retirement. You may think that you will plan what to do with your time nearer to retirement and flesh out the vague ideas you might have at that stage. Not a good idea, believe me. Personal reflection and planning are key!

What is of equal importance is to plan what to do with your time when all or most of the demands of work are no longer part of your life or feature as prominently. I have worked with many people over the years who are caught by the unexpected arrival of retirement or reduced working commitments and it can be traumatic if no thought and planning were given to what life beyond work might and could look like. Not planning ahead may mean that circumstances and events are foisted upon us rather than being in control of our lives post-career.

When planning for retirement, make sure to include reflections on balancing your own particular needs of fellowship and solitude. I reiterate my advice not to leave the planning too late. Someone like a personal coach could be a valuable resource to get you started and thinking about life beyond work and the adventures you could pursue if you chose to do so. As with anything else in life, it will be what you make of it. A reminder of what A represents in H.A.G.S., namely attitude. I leave you with a final thought, namely if you find yourself being lonely, take the initiative and seek groups, activities or volunteering that meet your needs of socialising.

The Fear of Ageing
and Depression

'Feelings are much like waves, we can't stop them from coming but we can choose which ones to surf.'

– Unknown

Fear comes in so many disguises. It goes without saying that every one of us will feel sad at some stage of our lives with painful events such as loss or long-term health problems triggering depression. However, depression and anxieties have become significant symptoms of modern society affecting people of all ages.

Depression at a later stage in life may be associated with a difficulty in letting go of the past and accepting that ageing is an inevitable and natural flow of life. I suggest that we often look back to our youth with rose-tinted glasses. As I mentioned in a previous chapter, realistically assess your experiences and recognise your youth wasn't necessarily all about the good old days and it came with its share of ups and downs.

It is also necessary to recognise that growing older does not guarantee a decline in health or the quality of life as portrayed by some of the stereotypes the media is fond of favouring. If we feel good about how we look and how we feel, we'll be much more open to new experiences, people and opportunities.

It's perfectly normal to have periods of feeling sad or anxious, especially if we are going through a difficult time. However, we need to be vigilant and not allow our fears to go unchecked as they may morph into depression and depression may creep up on us unnoticed. It is, therefore, important that we do a regular check of our internal state and sense of emotional wellbeing. Prevention, in this case, is so much healthier than the cure.

Feeling unable to cope and possibly struggling alone, may very well lead to depression. Depression will ultimately rob us of our enjoyment of life and make the simple things appear insurmountable. The downward spiral will continue, eroding our confidence and further making us feel even more inadequate pushing us down the slippery slope of depression.

It is true that depression is a common problem among older adults. However, I stress that it is by no means a normal part of ageing and needs to be put into context. In fact, studies show that the majority of older adults are actually more satisfied with their lives than younger people, despite having to manage more illnesses or physical problems. It is true that life changes will happen as we get older which may cause feelings of uneasiness, stress, and sadness.

It is worth bearing in mind that some physical health conditions may very well present themselves as depression. It may first and foremost be a health issue. When experiencing symptoms associated with depressions such as loss of sleep, appetite and fatigue, medical help and advice should be sought as the cause may be due to a physical condition rather than depression or anxiety.

Sometimes depression or anxiety can come out of the blue as was the case with my husband. We had spent a lovely Christmas with two of his children and their families, celebrating the New Year. Two days after the end of the festivities with everyone back to normal life, anxiety and depression hit him like a sledgehammer.

To this day, there is no obvious reason for this. My husband has always been cheerful and enjoyed life and overnight the person I thought I was married to had disappeared. It was like living with a stranger and no indication as to when my husband would return. It can be both frightening as well as challenging to the spouse of someone struggling with anxiety or depression. One feels totally helpless and impotent in dealing with it.

The symptoms my husband experienced were high levels of anxiety, not being able to settle for more than a few minutes and loss of appetite. Sleep was out of the question, making depression that much worse due to fatigue. He was tearful and unpredictable and could not tolerate the noise of any kind. He also avoided people including his family and found communication almost impossible. We enjoyed nothing more than discussing and debating any subject at length, but not during this period of depression and anxiety.

The most mundane daily activities became a major challenge. We got to know our GPs at the local surgery very well and our lives revolved around constant changes in medication and trying to find ways to support him in coping with the symptoms.

It was a very difficult year and no clear event that heralded the end of this challenging period. It was not a case of simply snapping out of it, but instead a gradual process. I have become hypersensitive to clues that might suggest a return of his depression, attempting to remove anything that might act as a trigger.

I can only speak from my own experience when I say as the partner of someone going through anxiety and depression, it is vital to take care of yourself so that you have the energy and resilience to support and be there for your partner. Whatever you do, seek help, even if your partner resists help from external sources. There is not a one-size-fits-all solution and it will be trial and error to find a combination of support strategies that will help them through the experience.

We are complex creatures and there will be an endless combination of factors or circumstances leading to depression, both physical as well as emotional. As I mentioned above, depression may very well be a symptom of other long-term physical illnesses. It may even be the consequences of a number of medications taking concurrently. In my husband's case, he has had undiagnosed health symptoms in excess of ten years that have significantly changed his quality of life. It will no doubt have been a contributing factor.

The journey with my husband has motivated me to try and find ways in which we can prevent depression from creeping up on us, especially as we get older. From my own experiences as well as the experiences of people with whom I have worked professionally over the years, I have come to recognise that we underestimate the impact of retirement on our lives and our general sense of wellbeing. Given the significance of retirement in our lives, I have dedicated a chapter on retirement. My advice once again is to plan for that eventuality.

Keeping busy with activities we enjoy and being physically active is critical in keeping depression at bay, especially if we have had a busy professional life. We are social creatures and interaction with others goes a long way in maintaining our mental wellbeing. I will stress throughout the book how important it is to maintain our health, both physical as well as mental. Refer to the foreword for the mnemonic of H.A.G.S. and what it stands for. However, you will also expect me to add that it is also within our power to do a great deal to ensure continued health.

The experience of depression in our mid-life is, in fact, a common occurrence throughout the world. Women appear to be more prone to depression than men or it may be that men are less willing to talk about their feelings.

Furthermore, it is important to bear in mind that for us women, the middle-life crisis is intricately bound up with transitions such as the peri-menopause, menopause, hormonal changes, retirement, empty nest syndrome and vitamin deficiencies to name but a few. Is it, therefore, any surprise that we may succumb to depression at some stage in our life as we get older?

Pursue a healthy lifestyle at all times and within your capabilities and budget. That means to eat healthy and nutritious meals. The whole ritual of preparing a meal, even if it is for one, can go a long way in fighting off depression. Due to our lifestyle, my husband and I often spend time apart and even when I am on my own, I continue to enjoy my ritual of preparing my evening meal.

I always play music, sometimes have a glass of wine, set the table and light the candles. I also enjoy creating colourful meals and buy the best ingredients I can afford. The result is a much more tasty, nutritious and enjoyable meal. It is so easy to have an endless supply of creative recipes, thanks to the Internet. So, get creative and avoid ready meals where and if possible!

The golden thread of this book is the power of our attitude. A healthy attitude results in resilience that helps us to cope with unexpected challenges that cross our paths. Getting up and being as active as you can will go a long way in lifting your sense of wellbeing. Volunteering and seeing the challenges others face will make us aware of our own blessings and as I've said in other chapters, an attitude of gratitude is a great antidote to depression.

Don't underestimate the supportive power of staying connected to your family and friends. Take the time to make new friends by becoming involved in various social or educational activities. Having friends and social connections mean there will be someone with whom you feel comfortable and able to share your worries and anxieties. A problem shared is a problem halved!

Having lived a number of decades with its myriad of experiences, life teaches us to become cautious. Fear creeps upon us as we grow up and age, curtailing our ability to be spontaneous and possibly even impulsive. However, it is imperative that we use logic and reason to assess these fears and challenge the perceived possible dangers that will probably never materialise. It's a fact of life that occasionally, we are dealt a bad hand, but our attitude will determine how we overcome such adversity and the lessons we take from the experience.

However, depression may be more than the sense of being unable to cope with whatever challenges you may face. I once again emphasise that depression is a common but serious mood disorder and if you are suffering, you need to consult with your GP and get the necessary help and support you need. Depression is a real illness with very real symptoms and is not a character flaw or means that you are weak in any way. It means you may need additional help over and above what I suggested earlier to manage depression.

Above all, be kind to yourselves and stop beating yourself up for not living up to an unrealistic image of yourself. We can do an awful lot for ourselves to keep the shadow of depression away from our door, but at times we need extra help.

I leave you with the idea of embracing whatever age you are and to be fearless beyond 50 as fear will stop you from pursuing your dreams and keep you a prisoner in the grey zone of conformity at best and contributing to depression at its worse.

Discovering Your Resilience

'It's your road and yours alone. Others may walk it with you, but no one can walk it for you.'

– Rumi

At some stage in all our lives, life unravels. Some of the challenges we will face have the ability to cut to the bone. We cling onto our resilience like the victims of a shipwreck would to a live raft. Losses or circumstances beyond our control may leave our hearts in shreds.

During such times, it is difficult to imagine that there is a light at the end of the tunnel. Nor does it seem possible that we would have the strength or resources to claw our way back to the top. To paraphrase Kafka, sometimes we need to throw our lives away in order to gain it. However, during the dark nights of the soul, it is very difficult to take comfort from these pearls of wisdom.

We know from experience that such moments, filled with intense despair, has the potential to provide us with the opportunity to befriend life by befriending ourselves at the deepest level. However, human life is incredibly resilient with many examples throughout history to testify to this fact.

Every living creature from the smallest insect to human beings experience fear at some point. Fear is often the result of facing the unknown or the perceived threat to our survival. However, fear could be seen as a tool to dismantle our old ways of being. It is during our darkest times that we discover our deepest strength. Often our pain and fear are the results of resisting the inevitable changing nature of life.

We are born, we grow old and we die. People and experiences come and go in our lives. Everything is always in the process of transition. The counterintuitive approach is to relax into the circumstances and not to resist or panic. It does not mean passivity, but acceptance instead. We can draw comfort from the fact that any experience, no matter how painful or destructive, is also in transition and will eventually pass.

According to one of the greatest philosophers, Friedrich Nietzsche, a fulfilling life requires embracing rather running away from difficulties. In a particularly emblematic selection from his notebook, he wishes on those who are important to him; suffering, desolation, sickness, ill-treatment and indignities. With friends like these, who needs enemies! However, what Nietzsche is trying to say is that these experiences demonstrate our worthiness by our ability to endure.

I do not wish such tortures upon you, but I also know that you will not escape your trials and tribulations. However, resilience gives us the means to cope and through openness and acceptance, we discover the support in whatever shape necessary when it matters the most.

During a recent walk on my local beach, I watched with fascination as a ship attempted to make its way into the safety of the harbour, listing dangerously as it did so. The seas were rough and it took a number of attempts before it succeeded. As I watched, I reflected on the lesson to be drawn from its determination and resilience to battle the stormy seas.

Like the ship, we need the resilience to make our way to a safe harbour where we can shelter from the storms. Such a harbour will be different things to different people. Maybe a good book, a hot cup of chocolate, tea, coffee, snuggled up in front of the TV with an old movie, a hot bath, yoga, meditation, mindfulness and many other options you can imagine.

Withdrawing from the world for short periods of time to take stock and recharge the batteries has the benefit of building and strengthening our resilience. Developing resilience is fundamental in helping us deal with the inevitable stormy seas we all face at times in our lives, whatever our age.

Resilience is not necessarily a trait we inherently have, but a process or a toolkit we can learn to develop. With older adults being the fastest-growing age group, it is important for us to understand the physical and psychological benefits of developing resilience. There is strong evidence to suggest that an optimistic frame of mind with the capacity for enjoyment goes a long way to develop resilience and contribute significantly to psychological wellbeing.

This is yet another area of research where science challenges the perceived frailty and lack of resilience in the older generation and suggests that we have the same or even greater capacity of developing resilience than the younger generation. Not only does resilience enable us to deal with life's challenges, but it also plays a critical role in longevity.

There is much research to remind us that our attitude towards life and our experiences makes a significant contribution to our ability to exercise the resilience muscle. It is also interesting to note that older women appear to have developed a higher level of resilience than men of the same age.

It may be attributed to experiences older women have had to deal with such as cultural and social changes, responsibilities for looking after a family and other caregiving and financial concerns. Women are seen as successful in nurturing social connections and building relationships with others, key ingredients in developing resilience as we age.

A resilient attitude is flexible in nature, allowing us to adapt to new or different circumstances. Cognitive behavioural psychology suggests that how we think about unpleasant events we encounter will largely determine our thoughts and behaviours towards such events. It is not the event itself, but our interpretation of it that will determine our emotions and reactions to certain situations and circumstances.

Research supports what I intuitively perceive, namely, that the effects of high resilience are linked to the quality of our lives, providing us with a greater sense of wellbeing both physically as well as mentally, enhancing longevity.

However, as with anything worth having, we have to work at it and taking time out to nurture ourselves is one of the many ways in which we can develop our resilience.

As I will say many times in different ways throughout this book, there is overriding evidence to suggest that lifestyle choices hugely contribute to our physical as well as psychological wellbeing, influencing our level of resilience. Therefore, taking the time out of busy schedules is critical in our ability to have the resilience to cope with the demands on our time and emotions.

We live in a society obsessed with doing, taking action and always striving to do better and more. Yet, it is vital to our physical and mental wellbeing to balance these activities with quiet times and self-care. There is a myriad of ways in which we can achieve this and each one of us needs to find our own safe harbour to shelter from the storms.

I certainly advocate a break away from technology and turning off tablets, smartphones, laptops and other electronic devices. Instead, do something different and take up yoga, meditation or mindfulness or at least go for a walk. I guarantee from experience that a walk in nature has a calming effect on a troubled mind. Another reminder of the mantra running through this book is the G in H.A.G.S., namely, get up and go! Every one of these letters, if practised, leads to resilience and wellbeing.

It is worth emphasising that resilience is mental as well as physical in nature. Both aspects of resilience result in a positive experience of ageing. An accepting view of growing older perceives ageing as a natural and continuous development of being human and not abnormal and to be avoided or resorting to feelings of guilt.

The relatively new discipline of neuroscience has gone a long way in dispelling some of the myths surrounding the so-called inevitable decline in old age. Brain plasticity, the quality of a substance to be shaped and moulded is associated with the flexibility of an organism to adapt and adjust to its environment. The discovery of such plasticity of the brain or neuroplasticity challenges the earlier beliefs that assumed the brain develops through childhood and then remains relatively unchanged.

Recent research findings of the plasticity of the brain suggest that it can be altered even in adulthood. The conclusion is that the brain is not hard-wired, but instead, our brains are capable of creating new pathways. The crunch is that this is influenced by our lifestyles, intellectual engagements, leisure activities and learning new skills.

One of the fascinating aspects of human nature that I have observed over the years is how some people not only overcome horrific experiences and adversity but actually seem to rise above these events and come out the other side much stronger. Instead of becoming bitter and disillusioned with life, they just get on with it. What makes them different from others, I wonder?

One example of such a person is Heather whom I had the privilege of meeting around the time my brother was on his journey with terminal cancer. Heather had already successfully overcome cancer on the left-hand side of her face, which had weakened the function of her eye and mouth muscles on that side. Fifteen years or so later, she was diagnosed with breast cancer and had to have a double mastectomy. There then followed months of radium and chemotherapy treatment and their debilitating side effects.

During this time, her attitude was always one of finding the positives of her ordeal, helping her to cope with the side-effects inflicted by the various treatments. Being a person that does not mince her words when confronted with young lads who taunted her for her appearance after losing her hair, she responded with a sharp reply, 'My excuse is cancer, what is yours?' Needless to say, even loutish lads were suitably embarrassed by their behaviour and comments.

The hospital staff often asked her to talk to other patients to comfort and encourage them with her positive attitude. After her treatment, she then had a number of years of regular follow-ups to check for any signs of cancer returning. It was only after she was given the all-clear that she was offered plastic surgery to reconstruct her breasts from fatty tissue taken from her abdomen.

It was not an easy procedure and once again she had to endure significant pain and infections. Alas, it was not successful and her body rejected the procedure. She refused another attempt and now proudly views her scarred torso and stomach as a reminder of being alive another day to pursue her interests with vigour and enthusiasm. Heather is an example of someone determined not to be governed by her circumstances, but to make the choice about her attitude and the way she would respond to the ordeals life placed in her path.

Thankfully, not all of us will experience what Heather had gone through. Nevertheless, we all face events and circumstances during our lifetime that challenge and test our ability to cope. What people like Heather remind us of is that there are constructive ways forward and always something to be grateful for, no matter how small.

Make the time to stop and enjoy the seasons, relishing in the small things and just enjoy the moment. I particularly savour the gift of calmness that ageing has brought. Seek out your safe harbour where you can shelter from the storms when they batter your shores, as they will from time to time.

An Antidote to Becoming a Grump

'Some people age like wine. Others age like milk.'
– Rebel Circus

It is our choice how we decide to age; wine or milk, at any given time in our life. I am not sure why society associates grumpiness with age, but it does. I challenge this assumption having had the displeasure of encountering grumpiness among the young as well as the old. However, given that it is connected with getting older I will explore what might lead to this unpleasant behaviour and hopefully advice on how to avoid becoming a grump at any age.

What are the tell-tale signs of a grumpy person and how can we recognise it in others and ourselves? Language is a good indicator of whether we are on the road to becoming grumpy. For example, the word 'too' should be seen as an early warning sign. It may be too cold, too hot, too noisy, etc. which seriously sounds like a moan. We also appear to have forgotten to smile or laugh. When was the last time you found something amusing or entertaining as opposed being irritated or annoyed by it? Not only does a good belly laugh make us feel much better, but you will also be delighted to hear that it consumes calories!

How often do we find ourselves complaining about the younger generation? It is unwarranted as the younger generation is probably a lot more tolerant of differences in others than the grumpy older person. Another warning sign is getting angry and resentful with the change, rejecting new ideas and objects without at least giving it a try before doing so.

We become entrenched in our comfort zones and have lost the sense of wonder, curiosity, excitement and willingness to embrace the unknown of our youth. We no longer experiment with the most elementary of things and prefer to do what we've always done. Why risk the unknown if we can stick with what we know and predict what we will get in return?

Gone is our sense of adventure. The consequences are that we deny ourselves the opportunity of new pleasures and the need for our minds to process new information, which, you will have read elsewhere, contributes to loss of our memories and agility of our brains.

Upgrades to the software are just one example that comes to mind. Yes, technology is constantly changing, which means we have to unlearn and relearn new ways of doing things all the time. No, there is not a conspiracy theory against the older generation. The inevitable changes following upgrades to various devices always result in my husband accusing a fictitious 'spotty youth' for creating change just to annoy customers. He does eventually come to accept the change and repeats the cycle with a new software upgrade. The bonus of changes such as these is that we are constantly learning which keeps our minds supple. View it as part of the mental gym for the brain.

My father was a firm believer that idleness leads to misdemeanours of all kinds and I think it is a truth to be applied at any age. Idleness, as we get older, will inevitably lead to depression, ill-health and heaven forbid, grumpiness. Reminder, the G in H.A.G.S. is get up and go and get moving!

Ageing, just as any aspect of life we have and will encounter, will be what we make of it. It is not just about loss but also about gains that come with ageing. As we get older, we gain wisdom and a deeper sense of who we are. We have many life experiences we can draw on to support us in dealing with what comes our way. Research confirms that we have a greater sense of gratitude as we get older, except perhaps for the grumps among us!

The research for my book brought me in contact with so many role models of what it is like to age with vigour and a passion for life. Many I met in person and others I came across as part of the research journey. One such woman I have not met personally but read about in numerous publications is a woman called Tao Porchon-Lynch, a yoga teacher at 97, a lover of wine and a competitive ballroom dancer who took up the latter at just age 80. She had her share of challenges but continued to pursue her passions despite having had three hip operations. I can hear the comments why it is not for you. I am too old to start, I have arthritis, I am alone…Fill in the blanks and keep a lookout for the examples of ordinary outstanding women and men I make reference to throughout the book. I also suggest that if you take a look around you at the people you encounter on a daily basis, you will find many of your examples of people who defy and rewrite the script of ageing.

It is not much fun being around a grumpy person and being one will inevitably result in isolation and loneliness. Who in their right mind would choose to spend time with a negative person who can only focus on what is wrong and annoying with the world as opposed to the positives in life? There are plenty of things to celebrate, if only we are willing to look for them.

However, all is not lost and recent research challenges the stereotype of the grumpy old man or women. Instead, it suggests that we actually become more tolerant and happier as we get older. It goes on to say that older people are also much more likely to be trusting of others than the younger generation.

There is significant research that suggests we become happier once we pass the 50+ mark. In fact, research concludes that we are at our happiest in our 60s, 70s, 80s and beyond. Just one of the many benefits of getting older, lest you forget that there are many benefits of ageing. It is also the age when we may not have to worry about climbing the career ladder. This allows us to live much more in the moment without having to chase unrealistic and ephemeral goals.

However, unfulfilled career aspirations may be the very reason why some people become grumpy as they harbour feelings of unrealised potential in their careers. Letting go of bitterness and frustrations such as these will go a long way in avoiding grumpiness and achieving a happier and more fulfilling existence.

As I pointed out above, it is true that there is a tendency to become set in our ways as we get older and the danger is that we lose our sense of adventure and therefore deny ourselves unexpected pleasures and experiences. It also contributes to grumpiness as we become averse to anything that challenges our predictable routine and an entrenched view of the world.

Yet again, science reminds us of the power of laughter, a powerful antidote to grumpiness. Having fun is not only for children and we are never too old to pursue what brings us joy. Laughter has been proved to have not only physical but positive psychological benefits. So, for your health and mental wellbeing, lighten up and see the funny side of life. Give yourself permission to go out and play and have some fun. If you are a grandparent, you have a ready-made excuse to be daft without feeling silly. The rest of us just need to draw on a bit more courage.

We must consciously challenge ourselves to step outside our comfort zones and to do at least one thing every day that we wouldn't normally do. Do you always shop on a Wednesday? How about Thursday instead? No, I hear you say, on Thursdays, we go for a coffee. Is there any reason why you cannot swop the days around or even go to the cinema instead of a coffee or both? Alternatively, make a point of looking at a familiar scene or event with new eyes as if seeing it for the first time. What have you not noticed before? Behind the comfort zones may lie a treasure chest of new experiences. Another workout as part of the mental gym for the brain. Be inventive!

It is true that life is not perfect, but as the A in H.A.G.S. remind us that we have the freedom to choose an attitude of acceptance when we are unable to change circumstances and events. A positive attitude will go a long way in helping us to accept what comes our way. I am once again reminded of the advice given by Mihaly Csikszentmihalyi in his book entitled, *The Flow*, suggesting activities that engender pleasure and lasting satisfaction are the sources of happiness.

Attitude is a mindset; a choice that has a significant impact on the quality of our daily living. If we want to change our lives the options are in the first instance that life and circumstances have to change or secondly, we are the ones who need to do the changing. Often the latter is what brings about long-term, sustainable change. It also results in a lot less bruises! I dedicate a chapter to the benefits of a positive attitude, but as a reminder, our quality of life is significantly impacted by the attitude with which we approach the experience of our lives.

I want to propose an antidote to grumpiness. Have you ever heard the saying, 'act your age, not your shoe size?' This saying is normally meant as a rebuke as the person it is aimed at is presumed to behave in a childish manner. I pose a counter-argument to say acting your shoe size more often will prevent the slide into grumpiness. Let me explain.

If you are a U.K. size 5, 6 or 7 say, cast your mind back to who you were at that age. How did you view the world? How did you behave? It is an age when we are insatiably curious seeking answers to the many things that baffled us. I recall my father saying to me with exasperation after endless 'whys' that he was not a walking encyclopaedia. We are filled with uncensored imagination and playfulness.

We have boundless energy and express creativity in many ways. Time was of no concern to us and we lived in the moment, expressing the flow I made reference to earlier. How does that compare to the person we have become over the years, stressing about lack of time, curtailing our spontaneity and often our imaginations, dismissing it as immature. We are much less willing to take risks and following our curiosity and enthusiasm. Curiosity ensures we keep on learning and discovering new things as well as new ways of doing things.

Margo is a prime example and shared her excitement with me of learning the art of managing olives, pruning, picking and pressing and everything else necessary in producing olive oil. Apart from managing their olive grove, she relishes being a fun grandma and embracing her inner child. She just loves playing and entering the world of make-believe. I have no doubt that she is a grandma any child would want to spend time with, irrespective of her age. Her grandchildren will carry with them the treasured memories of fun times spent with their youthful grandmother.

It is within our power to reignite these behaviours within ourselves. We can once again cultivate more positive approaches to life. Laughter at our shoe size was always just below the surface, ready to breakthrough. Practice to view things in a more light-hearted way and find reasons to laugh more often. Not only does it have a positive impact on our lives, but it also brings people together, friends, family and strangers.

You have had to live on another planet not to have encountered the discussions about mindfulness and living more mindfully. It is a positive strategy especially for our distracted modern life that allows us to once again enjoy even the simple things in life in the moment and without distraction. We are always where we are and where we need to be. Enjoy the moment.

I, therefore, categorically encourage you to act your shoe size more often to once again experience the wonder, joy and light-heartedness of your younger self. She is in there somewhere; all you have to do is invite her back into your life.

The conclusion is yes, our personalities change as we get older. However, there is no scientific evidence to suggest that we necessarily become grumpy and angry with the world as we get older. Nor do we need to collude with the stereotype of being a grumpy older person. Grumpiness may have more to do with our personalities than a fact of ageing. It is, therefore, up to us to guard against emotional sloppiness and exercise a positive attitude of gratitude for our blessings. The choice is ours, so choose wisely.

Letting Go

'The woman who follows the crowd will usually not go
further than the crowd. The woman who walks alone is likely
to find herself in places no one has ever been before.'

– Albert Einstein

The following simple but powerful story brought home to
me how destructive hanging on to the past can be. It also made
me realise that we alone have the power to do something
about it.

Two monks were on a pilgrimage. One day, they came to
a deep river. At the edge of the river, a young woman sat
weeping because she was afraid to cross the river without
help. She begged the two monks to help her. The younger
monk turned his back. The members of their order were
forbidden to touch a woman.

But the older monk picked up the woman without a word
and carried her across the river. He put her down on the far
side and continued his journey. The younger monk came after
him, scolding him and berating him for breaking his vows. He
went on this way for a long time.

Finally, at the end of the day, the older monk turned to the
younger one. 'I only carried her across the river. You have
been carrying her all day.'

Just as with the younger monk, we continue to carry the
burden of our past with us all day long, often at tremendous
cost. However, letting go is difficult and we all have a long
list of things we find challenging to leave in the past where it
belongs. The list will range from habits, beliefs, ideas,
assumptions, through to destructive relationships, guilt,
resentment and so much more besides.

Just as with physical clutter, mental and emotional clutter elbows out any possibility of new experiences. If unchecked, our obsession with the past will become our prison. The sad thing is that the present will pass us by and we may lose what is really important in our lives.

Not only does the inability to let go affect our own lives, but it also affects the lives of those around us, particularly the people closest to us. Our burden becomes their burden and we inadvertently damage or destroy our relationships with others by refusing to let go of the past.

In my experience working as a coach over years, some of my clients needed support in struggling with pending retirement. They found it difficult to make the transition due to their inability to let go of the professional lives they have lived and everything associated with it. For so many years, they have confused their identities with their job title. It came as a surprise to Françoise reflecting on all the challenges she had to cope with during her 40s and 50s and how much easier life was if you allowed it to happen rather than trying to control it.

Continuing with her reflections, now in her 70s, Françoise concludes just how much the commitment to learning and being open to different perspectives has made a difference to her journey after retirement. For her, it was a total growth path and not wasting one of the precious years in her later life. Each year, she has done something that has made her a bigger and better person. She now feels that at this stage in her life, her next growth has to be in giving back to society and her community in some way.

Although we recognise intellectually that letting go is the first step in embracing a new life, accepting it emotionally and living it are two very different things. Tactics such as avoidance and procrastination will only make it worse. Tracey shared with me how she came to realise just how much her career had dominated her thoughts and waking moments. It was when she felt overwhelmed and unable to get the rest her body yearned for that she said enough was enough. She negotiated a part-time contract with her employer and now works only three days a week. It has made a significant difference to her quality of life. Her only regret was that she didn't have the confidence to make a career change much earlier in her life.

Apart from letting go of a demanding career, Tracey has also come to value herself and her needs and as she says she is no longer prepared to be the peacekeeper in the family and bending backwards to keep everyone happy. She has learnt to say 'no' at all levels of her life and is much happier for it. Furthermore, Tracey gained in confidence to challenge the assumptions others had of her and her needs.

Her husband had retired before her and one of the assumptions was that she will follow suit and retire to spend time with her husband instead of wanting to continue working. This assumption was accompanied by one that suggested that surely, she was now too old to start new adventures and pursuing opportunities, working freelance for herself or even the not so hidden message that it was perhaps indulgent to pursue new ventures. Tracey's experience is not unique and many women face criticism and surprise when in later life they decide to dust off the cobwebs from their dreams and, being free of caring and possibly career responsibilities, pursue their dreams with vigour and passion.

Reflecting on our experiences and resistance helps us to gain awareness and insight into what we need to do in order to break the cycle. It is worth recognising that we are not our past experiences and circumstances, nor our thoughts. We have the power to walk away from those experiences intact. They do not define who we are. Tracey reflected that giving up the need to always do the right thing and feeling compelled to compete with others, gave her the freedom and permission to take a step back and design the life that suited her and meet her personal needs.

The things we hang on to often provide us with a reward or payback, even if it is negative in nature. Reflection can go a long way in understanding what the benefits might be and how we can find what we need in other more positive ways.

In order to create and embrace a new future with new experiences, we have to first let go of the old to make room for the new to enter. The first step is to accept the past for what it is. We cannot go back and rewrite history, but we have the choice to move on, no matter how difficult it may seem.

It is apparent from the stories women have shared with me that one of the things many of them have had to let go of is the need to please and to put the needs of others before their own. I can relate to this as well and have spent most of my life feeling guilty for what I wanted or didn't want, especially if it was in conflict with the needs of others. The society I grew up in also instilled perhaps unhealthy respect for authority that meant I could never say no to the demands of the organisation or my superiors. Our society also explicitly advocated that the needs of men came before women. Add all of that together and putting my needs first or even considering doing so was very difficult and impossible most of the time.

These words resonate with Vanessa and the sense of independence she gained as she got older. She now has the confidence of being able to present herself as the person she is and not being overly concerned about what others think of her body, clothes and opinions.

It is only now at the age of 60+ that I am very comfortable to include my own needs and wants into the discussions and negotiations whether at a personal or professional level. Jetting the burden of pleasing others at a cost to my own needs has probably been one of the most liberating and rewarding experiences of getting older.

I feel like an excited child again now that I am comfortable in revisiting dreams and experiences I yearned to explore over the years. I, therefore, encourage you to consider whether a more balanced and healthier inclusion of your needs as well would also benefit your sense of wellbeing. Furthermore, what I have also gained is greater respect from others who recognise that I am equally entitled to realising my own needs instead of subjecting them to the demands and whims of others.

Letting go of emotional baggage is very challenging and it is easy to get caught up in a downward spiral and convince ourselves that there is no way out. The walls of our prison seem impossible to scale. Yet, there is always a hidden exit, just persevere and the support of a friend or a confidante may provide the key to unlock the escape route.

Some let go of demanding careers and embark on adventures and pursuing their dreams. Veronica had a very demanding career as a director working in a stressful environment within the charity sector. At the age of 50, she and her husband decided to rethink a busy and stressful life and to pursue their lifelong dream to move to France. That is precisely what they did and have never looked back. They embraced the culture, the language and the people with open hearts and a willingness to immerse themselves into the French culture. Veronica confirms they have no regrets and despite coping with the challenges of living in a different culture, trying to navigate bureaucracy in a different language, it was worth every minute.

I will add that both Veronica and her husband were willing to flex, adapt and embraced the whole experience with open minds and with an attitude of gratitude that they were in a position to pursue their dreams. Others I have met who may have done the same and moved to another country were not as complementary to the host country and their attitude probably had a lot to do with it. It comes as no surprise that having a sense of entitlement and expecting the host culture to adapt to your cultural ways is going to lead to disappointment.

Psychology and counselling advocate the need to examine our past in order to embrace the future. However, there comes a point when continued pontification of the past becomes quicksand from which it is difficult to extricate ourselves.

It requires effort on our part and a willingness to take action alongside reflecting on past experiences. An effort is necessary to get past our human reluctance to change. We are creatures of habit even if the habit inflicts pain. Be prepared to come up with compelling and distorted reasons for clinging to the status quo, driven by our fear of the unknown.

At some point, we also have to acknowledge and recognise the contribution we have made to past hurts or failures. Taking our share of responsibility for past events gives us the power to choose the present and create a new future. Being the victim keeps us firmly rooted in the past. It also denies us the opportunity to a much more rewarding future.

I have always been a believer that having a good clear out paves the way for new things to take the place of the old. It can apply to the clearing out of physical objects or a mental clear out. This could include old beliefs, habits, etc. that are no longer relevant in our lives or make a positive contribution.

The 'old' could represent our comfort zones, a place where we may feel safe and secure, representing predictability and stability. However, such a place may very well prevent us from experiencing new situations and adventures and in time may become a prison without us realising it. Furthermore, clutter spreads into other areas of our lives. Clutter equals stress.

I acknowledge having a clear-out is easier said than done. Most of us procrastinate and sometimes for years before we get around to throwing out the old, even if it was in our best interest to have done so a long time ago. Coupled with procrastination might be a sentimental attachment to the physical, mental or emotional things we need to let go of. We might cling on to our clutter for dear life just like a child with a comfort blanket. It could, of course, be sheer laziness preventing us from doing what needs doing.

However, when we eventually get around to the clear out, it is a very rewarding and cathartic experience. It is as though a physical weight has been lifted off our shoulders, accompanied by a sense of wellbeing or even euphoria. A saying that will be familiar to most of us, namely 'if you do what you've always done, you will get what you've always got', offers some insight into the benefit of ridding ourselves of the old.

The Chinese philosophical system of feng shui refers to the flow of energy in our lives, both physical and mental and advocates the free-flowing of energies in and through our lives. Ridding ourselves of physical and mental barriers enables positive energy to flow more freely.

My mantra has always been that if I haven't used something or worn a piece of clothing for a year, it is time to get rid and that includes our digital lives. Be ruthless with emails, mailing lists and information that are no longer relevant.

I have mentioned a number of times in previous chapters that preparation for retirement is critical to a positive experience. The notion of a good clear out of both physical and mental clutter is a significantly powerful act in the preparation of embracing either part-time or full-time retirement. Old habits, beliefs and actions may no longer be relevant and in order to embrace and benefit from new experiences, changes are critical.

It is the perfect time to rid us of both physical and mental clutter that no longer have any benefit in our lives. In doing so, we successfully pave the way for a different life, making way for new experiences and adventures. The process of doing so can be an emotional experience and there is no need to do it all at once. You now have the time to do what you have always put off doing in the past.

That is exactly what I have been doing a few months after I took semi-retirement. I realised that my large wardrobe of business clothing represented a professional identity that no longer catered for my new lifestyle and persona. It took quite some time for me to let go of clothing I was very fond of but doing so allowed me to enjoy experimenting with new informal styles and colours that I would have considered inappropriate for a professional environment.

The added benefit was that not only did I enjoy the journey of creating a more relevant wardrobe, but it also allowed me to de-clutter my emotional wardrobe as well. I took a hard look at the habits and beliefs I had about myself and cleared out those that were irrelevant, allowing me to embrace new aspects of myself.

So, be brave and make time for a spring clean, irrespective of the time of year, in order to make room for the new!

Midlife Crisis
The Time to Dream

'You are never too old to set another goal or dream a new dream.'

– C. S. Lewis

Many of us assume that when we are near or enter retirement, it also means giving up on unfulfilled dreams and desires. However, Lewis reminds us that age has nothing to do with it. Age is not a barrier and merely an excuse. Be careful of the stories you tell yourself as they may lead to self-fulfilling prophecies.

For example, everyone knows that as we get older, the decline of both our bodies and our minds is inevitable. Life may also become less satisfying and enjoyable. It is also a time that there may be cognitive decline associated with ageing and inevitably we may become less productive at work.

I bet you've been nodding your head in agreement and guess what, think again because you are wrong! Studies over recent years have challenged many of the myths surrounding ageing.

Myth number 1: Depression is more prevalent in old age.

I discussed depression at length in an earlier chapter. There is, however, an assumption that there is an inevitable decline of general health as we age. This means it will, therefore, be difficult to maintain a positive outlook on life.

However, research indicates that emotional well-being continues to improve until our 70s when it begins to level off.

Contrary to the belief that youth represents the best time of our lives, the peak of emotional life may very well occur when we are in our 70s and beyond. As we get older, we tend to focus more on the positive than the negative.

Myth number 2: Cognitive decline is inevitable.

Our older brains behave a bit like an older computer, which means that it takes longer to process and retrieve information from the huge bank of memories we have built up over the years. The fact that knowledge and experience increase with age, older adults, therefore, do better when tested in the real world than when tested in laboratories.

Study after study proves again and again that learning new skills improves our memories. I touch on this subject in a number of chapters but given its importance and significance, I will remind you about it periodically.

Myth number 3: Older workers are less productive.

Thanks to the stereotype that suggests older workers are less adaptable than younger workers, they are also perceived as less productive. Once again studies have shown there is almost no relationship between age and performance in the workplace. On the contrary, jobs that require experience means older adults have the edge. They also tend to offer more loyalty than their younger counterparts.

Myth number 4: Loneliness is more likely.

In a number of chapters, I share research findings of the importance of well-being and our social connections with others. Studies also suggest that older adults have closer ties with members of their social networks than those of younger adults. It would appear that on average older adults are less lonely than young people. One reason may be that we have more time to devote to relationships. We are also of a generation that did not grow up with social media and therefore our interactions with people have been in person or via telephone.

Myth number 5: Creativity declines with age.

The assumption has always been that creativity is the province of the young. However, studies have proved that it is during midlife when artists and scholars are at their most prolific. This is particularly true in fields that require accumulated knowledge.

Conceptual artists tend to produce their best work in their 20s and 30s whereas experimental artists reach their full potential later in life. Like good wine, the latter improves with age and experience. Michael Angelo designed the Dome of St. Peters when in his 90s and Picasso painted for most of his 91 years. So, the list goes on.

Myth number 6: More exercise is better.

The G in H.A.G.S. reminds us that exercise is key to improving health and longevity. However, there is growing evidence to suggest that more is not necessarily better. There is a point of diminishing returns. Exercising for health is different from exercising for fitness. Doing a bit every day is better than a burst once or twice a week.

It would appear that long-term strenuous endurance exercise may actually cause 'overuse injury' to the heart. The message once again confirms that a regular but moderate cardiovascular workout, such as a good brisk walk, is much better than vigorous daily exercise.

Of course, there are certain things we can't control or influence as part of the ageing process. However, we have absolute control over creating self-fulfilling prophecies of what our life might look like in later years.

Our self-perceptions about ageing influence our thoughts and behaviours without us consciously being aware of this. If they are of a negative nature, it will ultimately lead to collusion with the myths set out above.

We live in interesting times marked by a strong sense of uncertainty and unpredictability. It seems as though the rules are being rewritten on all fronts. At the time of writing, we are experiencing a change in the international political arena, the likes of which we haven't seen for generations. However, with change often come opportunities and a new order of things.

Yet the fear of the unknown has the power to paralyse us in the present, pushing away our hopes and dreams. Our logical mind chastises us for our fears as it is impossible to predict what may occur in the future. Instead of enjoying the here and now, our fears rob us of the present as we get caught in the web of a hypothetical future with all its doom and gloom.

Fear comes in so many disguises and a powerful fear is that of standing out and defying the norms and expectations as dictated by society. We feel uncomfortable to go against the flow and will often keep silent rather than be the odd one out. I was reminded recently of exactly that.

Having more time on my hands, I have been on a mission to redecorate a number of rooms in my house. Contemplating colour schemes for my kitchen, my instinct was to be bold and go for strong colours. I immediately felt the fear of non-conformity and what the reaction of others might be. Anyone who knows me will testify that I am very comfortable with going against the norm. Yet, here I was reacting to a fear of rejection and possible criticism of my non-conventional taste.

Our social conditioning is very strong and capable of suppressing the playful child within us. As we get older, that voice is ever-present to remind us of how we should behave, what we can and can't do, what we should and shouldn't wear and what society expects of us as the older generation. Not to mention all the doom and gloom associated with getting older.

We begin to fear the decline of our physical as well as our mental health and what we consider to be the inevitable constraints on what we might be capable of doing in the future. The ultimate fear, of course, is death. There is a balance between accepting that with getting older, our bodies require different treatment versus giving up on playfulness, optimism and the enjoyment of a new phase of life.

From personal experience, our 50s is a critical time for us to learn to deal with the fear of getting older. We have a foot in both camps. We are not in the flush of youth, yet we are not what we might consider a senior citizen. It is, therefore, the perfect time to deal with the unrealistic fear of getting older and to tame the beast before it deprives us of our dreams and enjoyments of a life beyond the daily toil of earning a living.

Ageing can be particularly daunting to women. Given the messages we receive throughout our lives in terms of our appearance, the fear of getting older looms large and menacing. We fear the loss of our looks and the gravitational pull, which will inevitably result in saggy breasts, wrinkles, dry skin, possible weight gain, the inability of gracefully teetering around in stilettos and worst of all, becoming invisible.

It is also a time when women go through significant changes, namely the menopause. In fact, the final myth is that it isn't merely a 'change', but a transition. It is not something that happens to us overnight and you are not going to wake up one morning and be in the grip of hot flushes, mushy minds and emotions that are dragging you around a rollercoaster ride. Granted, although it is a gradual transition, the symptoms will sometimes feel immediate and like bolts out of the blue.

Remember, all of these symptoms are real as is the transition you are going through. However, don't suffer in silence and seek help if you feel you need it. At least share your experience and symptoms with your family, friends and in particular, your significant other. Stoic is good, but suffering unnecessarily when help is available is being masochistic. Pre-empting what some of you may be thinking, there is absolutely nothing to be ashamed of as it is a very natural part of the journey of being a woman.

This journey too will come to pass. The benefits are that it is time for recalibration. We re-evaluate life and relationships and are no longer willing to be put upon, tolerate abuse or being disrespected. We recognise that we do not need to contort ourselves into shapes Houdini would have been proud of. It is a time when we truly begin to celebrate our strengths and gracefully accept our weaknesses without the need to beat ourselves up about it. More about the menopause in the following chapter.

At this time of our lives, we begin to recognise the media mantra of having to chase the elusive fountain of eternal youth for what it is. If like me you've coloured your hair, you begin to embrace the idea of going grey and discovering your hair for what it really is. We have the courage to explore with wearing what pleases us whether it is labelled suitable for our age or not because we can. No, this is not letting ourselves go, but instead, we are embracing and celebrating the beauty of who we are at this stage and age of our lives. We step through a portal into selfhood and self-confidence.

Not only do we acquire wisdom with age, but we also accumulate more memories of past failures and as a result, we may hold back on our dreams. We may also become jaded and wary thereby less likely to take chances in case we fall short of our expectations.

It is so easy to give up on longings and activities we didn't have the time or opportunity to pursue during the years of earning a living and bringing up a family. We may also feel slightly embarrassed, wondering what others may think if we take up a particular activity or pursuit at a later stage in life.

A lot of energy goes into suppressing the whispering of our longings and unfulfilled dreams, justifying why it would be ridiculous and silly to do so at this stage of life. Instead, all of that energy could be harnessed into pursuing our dreams, throwing caution to the wind.

So, what if your friends and acquaintances think you're going through a mid-life transition and yes, you may very well fail and realise that it didn't provide the reward and fulfilment you always thought it would. On the other hand, it might just bring unexpected rewards to your life and the only way to find out is to give it a go.

Challenging the ageism all around us is not only for ourselves but for future older women as well. It is our duty. This includes challenging the mantra that assumes every woman wants to remain eternally youthful and stop the clock of ageing as if it is within anyone's ability to do. Be vigilant and conscious of slipping into the trap of using ageist language and challenge the stereotypes of ageing where and whenever possible.

Don't be tempted to blame everything on your age, such as a lapse of memory being labelled as a 'senior moment'. Young people are forgetful as well and it is not the privilege of the older generation. There are so many positives about ageing as I discuss throughout the book, focus on these rather than the negatives.

Again, a reminder that the A in H.A.G.S. is for attitude and that means embracing and accepting your older self. Doing so does not mean we give up and automatically join a faceless homogenous and invisible group in society. It is also not an excuse for resisting the yearning to pursue different interests and activities. Yes, I know, it takes confidence to go against the tide.

However, the key to feeling confident about ourselves is to value who we are. I also know that it will be a big ask for some of you. So, start small and allow it to grow in momentum. If others are going to value us, we need to start with valuing ourselves. Feeling good about the woman in the mirror begins with our grooming and taking care of our appearance, hence the importance of clothing, makeup and hairstyle. I devote much discussion on this topic throughout the book, supported with practical examples and tips.

We underestimate the power of language to influence how we feel about ourselves. So, pay attention to the language you use when referring to yourself. Are you always putting yourself down? Why not begin by acknowledging your strengths and good points instead. No, you're not too old to start something totally new. Value your own opinion. You've been around long enough to have developed a valid point of view about many topics. Start taking care of yourself not only as far as your appearance goes, but your diet, health and exercise regime. The saying 'behave as if' is so true; act with confidence and that you matter and eventually, your mindset and behaviour will follow.

I return to the myths and stories I discussed in a previous chapter and it is understandable why women at a later stage of their lives were seen as a threat by the patriarchy. They began to challenge oppressiveness where they found it; they spoke out for the weak and because of it were labelled heretics and witches and burnt at the stake. In different ways, we are still resisting those forces trying to tell us what we should look like as we get older, how we should behave, what we should and shouldn't wear, etc., etc. Embrace your journey to cronehood and proudly wear your crown of wisdom with grace.

It takes courage to give ourselves permission to take the first step in pursuing our unfulfilled passions. It is also difficult to silence the ever-present voice of the critical parent in our heads no matter how old we are. Your parents no doubt suppressed their own dreams and longings. As a result, they may have encouraged or insisted that you pursue a proper job with the perceived security that goes with it.

In my case, my father had a strong belief in the power of education. On the other hand, my interests and rewards came from artistic pursuits. These two belief systems were in conflict and the result was that I was channelled into an education dominated by the sciences and mathematical subjects. Not only did these subjects not provide me with any fulfilment, but I also struggled in grasping to understand what they were all about.

In time, I managed to find a way of shaping my education to provide me with personal fulfilment in my career, but deep down, I continued to long for my first love of creativity, design and colour. It has taken me more than two years to finally give myself permission to carefully open the padlocked box that contains my unfulfilled dreams and desires.

Slowly, I am taking the time to reacquaint myself with my unfulfilled passions and also to allow them to be expressed in a way with the forms and shapes that reflect the person I have grown into over the years. I am also aware that they will change and go in directions I am not able to envisage at the moment and that is part of the excitement of the unknown.

Who knows what shape and personality my experiments will eventually assume? I am enjoying the journey of discovery without trying to anticipate or control what the outcome should be. I can now indulge in creative activities without the need for an end goal to be achieved within a particular time frame. Instead, I am allowing them the space to emerge and take the form they need to be. And guess what? The skies haven't fallen in yet!

So, what are the unfulfilled dreams and passions that you have nurtured over the years? More importantly, what are you denying the world by giving up on your dreams and secret longings? Is now perhaps your time too?

The Change

'People may call what happens at midlife 'a crisis,' but it is not. It's an unravelling – a time when you feel a desperate pull to live the life you want to live, not the one you're 'supposed' to live... to let go of who you think you are supposed to be and to embrace who you are.'

– Brené Brown

The first thing to remember about the menopause is that it is not 'the change' as it is so often referred to. Instead, it is a transition, or a rite of passage, which happens over a period and with a number of stages along the journey. As with any journey, it is likely to be different from one woman to another as we are all unique individuals. However, there may be similarities and experiences others have had that may be useful to us on our journey. Officially, we enter menopause approximately 12 months after our last period with the run-up to it identified as the peri-menopause. The duration of both stages will vary from woman to woman.

Every one of us will experience the journey through hot flushes, irregular and missed periods, sweating, shivers, possible depression, sleepless nights, sexual issues and back to hot flushes in our own unique way. Sounds depressing, doesn't it? As with life in general, our journey through this transition is personal to each of us. We will experience the same symptoms, but in fits and starts and severity each in our own way. And one final kick, it can last for years!

It is also not unusual for our lives to come under scrutiny as a result of the menopause, often as a consequence of hormonal changes and the effects on our brains. For example, we may be more willing to challenge and speak out against what we may perceive as injustices as well as discovering hidden wisdom and insight. Creativity is also given a new lease of life, rekindling desires and longings locked away for long periods of time. It is therefore understandable why it may have become known as 'the change'.

As Christiane Northrup suggests, continuing to suppress these desires and urges may very well lead to ill health. During this stage of rebalancing, you may very well resort to some uncharacteristic behaviour and expression of emotions to the surprise and shock of your nearest and dearest. In time we learn to articulate our needs and opinions in a more balanced and effective way. Remember the days of PMS?

One thing all women will all have in common is that the menopause marks a time for growth and expansion. It is also a time for re-evaluation and rebalancing of our priorities and an emphasis on quality over quantity. You may also begin to put yourself and your wellbeing at the top of the priority list where it belongs. It is also the time to experiment with a new and updated image to reflect who you are and the person you are rediscovering.

My personal experience reflects what Christiane Northrup writes about in her books, namely the willingness to speak up and challenge in a way we may not have had before. I mentioned that I was brought up in a culture where authority wasn't questioned and inevitably came in the shape of a man or men. My father was a very strong character and I never dared challenge or question his authority. This spilt over into my professional and personal lives and the socialisation from the minute I opened my eyes told me, that as a girl, I had to be nice, pretty and not brash in order to be liked.

My voice was silenced or tempered in most areas of my life and it is true that during the menopause period, I came out and stood my ground. I remember so clearly the day I finally challenged my father's authority and pushed back strongly. I don't know who was more surprised and shocked; me or my father! It was long overdue and I also think my father respected me for it. My need to being heard and to pursue long lost desires and ambitions has permeated all aspects of my life and I am now very comfortable with being kind to myself and exercise some self-love as well rather than always put others first at the expense of my own desires and needs. The message is that we need to be conscious of the fact that many things in our lives may shift, especially our relationships with others.

Many women refer to mushy brains and severe memory loss, forgetting names of people they have known forever or of places that have played a big role in their lives. I have been known to forget the names of colleagues I had worked with for more than 10 years, much to my embarrassment. Some women fear they may have early onset of dementia. These were the experiences of a number of women I interviewed, especially that of Margarette. She identifies the peri-menopause as a worrying time for her. She had always enjoyed excellent health and was therefore alarmed to notice a number of symptoms, especially loss of short-term memory function. With a lack of publicly available information or advice, she tried to ignore a growing concern that she may be in the early stages of Alzheimer's.

Finally, Margarette consulted a doctor when she began to have hot flushes at work and her relief was huge to have the diagnosis that she was in the early stages of the menopause. Her symptoms were the result of the normal consequences to be expected during this time. Understanding what was happening helped her in managing her response to her symptoms.

A number of women shared with me a critical aspect of going through the menopause, namely, that it was not possible for them to disclose any of their experiences in their professional environment and the need to hide it. The age at which women go through the menopause means they are often at a fairly senior level of the organisation, juggling stressful jobs alongside family commitments and then also having to deal with menopausal symptoms. The majority of women will avoid disclosing the challenges and symptoms they are experiencing with colleagues or their line manager.

The symptoms can be challenging at the best of times, but especially having to manage these within a work context.

Dealing with heavy periods, hot flushes and mushy brains, not to mention the mood swings pose additional stress in an already stressful life. Then there are the night sweats irrespective of the seasons and the volcanic eruptions of hot flushes that overwhelm you leaving you looking like an overripe tomato.

As I mentioned above, be prepared for the menopause to have a significant impact on your life on all levels. Vanessa, a normally optimistic, confident and outgoing woman, suffered from anxiety and sleeplessness. In addition, she was very wound up, emotional and lost the self-confidence she had previously possessed. Finally, in her 60s, she feels so much calmer, happier, positive, confident, contented, self-respectful and loves herself again. It is the time in between that is challenging for working women.

Tracey had similar experiences to that of Vanessa. She identified the peri-menopause as physically awful, which continued during the menopause. For her, it was difficult to manage at times with heavy periods and as so many of us experience, lack of sleep and general 'fuzziness'. She also became very moody and irrational at times. Tracey also went through periods of intense emotions, feeling a terrible sense of loss and anxiety related to her daughters as they were in their teenage years and testing the boundaries. Furthermore, Tracey didn't feel understood by anyone. I can very well imagine the challenges of coping with your own hormonal changes, let alone those experienced by teenage daughters. Difficult to say the least!

Thankfully, as with most of us, the post-menopause for Tracey brought a sense of freedom from the symptoms, being calmer and rejuvenated, but also a sense of limbo to a certain extent, accompanied by low libido, not an uncommon experience for women during or after the menopause as a result of a decline in hormones. The symptoms are a decrease in sex drive as well as vaginal dryness resulting in painful sex, leading to a further decline of the sex drive. There are numerous solutions to combat low libido and once again, your GP is the best person to discuss this with in the first instance.

It is worth mentioning that sex is not the only way to maintain intimacy with your partner. Be open and discuss the issues and together find a solution that works for both of you.

Although the menopause is still a taboo subject that is referred to only behind closed doors, there is increasing help available. The most obvious is HRT and it is a subject to explore with your medical practitioner particularly in the light of the waxing and waning of research associated with it. Make an informed decision whether it is for you or whether you prefer to go the alternative route, supported by supplements, acupuncture, diet or other options.

Although it is just one other natural cycle that we as women will experience. It is worth reflecting on the fact that we are likely to live on average thirty or more years beyond the menopause. It is therefore a time to appreciate the changes we will go through and what we can do to ensure life beyond the menopause will be a healthy and happy one. As you would expect, I am once again going to remind you to stay active. Our hormones are not the only thing that impacts the quality of our lives, our lifestyles are equally as significant, if not more so.

The International Menopause Society confirms the role lifestyle plays in minimising the symptoms of menopause. It includes eating a nutritious and healthy diet, especially if we may be prone to middle-age spread during this time. Another motivating reason to stay or become as active as possible. The IMS supported by numerous other researches suggest that women who are inactive are likely to experience more severe symptoms of menopause than women who remain active.

During and after the menopause, we become prone to osteoporosis and exercise and a healthy diet are two of the most significant factors contributing to healthy bones. Now is also the time to consider including vitamin and other supplements but check with your GP before doing so as a healthy diet should be the best place for us to access all the nutrients we need.

Yes, it is true that research once again supports the power of attitude and suggests that viewing this stage of our life with a positive and accepting attitude can and do make a difference to the way we experience the associated symptoms. A study by the Mayo Clinic suggests that practising mindfulness during the menopause may ease depression, anxiety and other emotional symptoms. There is a plethora of articles, blogs and books available that offer support. Sound research reinforces the benefits of mindfulness and meditation at all ages, but particularly as we grow older. The menopause stage is no different and it goes a long way in reducing stress and improve our overall health and wellbeing.

I sense the waves of resistance as you are reading this. Another activity to add to a very long list of demands that face you on a daily basis. I guarantee this is one activity worthy of taking the time to practice. It will give you the tools and state of mind to deal with the rest of the challenges you have to deal with for the remainder of the day. It is your choice whether to get up just 15 minutes earlier when the household is still quiet and practice some self-love or taking 15 minutes or more at the end of the day to destress before going to bed. It will be one of the best decisions you have ever made. Trust me!

In the resources section, I have included a number of authors who have written with authority, in my opinion, about the menopause, symptoms and practical solutions to these. Trust your curiosity and instincts and explore the various resources that may benefit you during not only the menopause but towards the journey of ageing positively.

It is also the time to revisit your beauty regime and your wardrobe as these things go a long way in making us feel good about ourselves and boosting our confidence. I have spoken about the added benefits of personal grooming to looking our best at length in another chapter. It is essential to look after ourselves, our skins and our minds and the effort is worth every minute, I assure you. As with mindfulness, pampering yourself is not an indulgence, it is essential maintenance. It also contributes greatly to supporting a zest for life!

The overarching message is, don't suffer in silence as there is a lot of help and support out there, starting with your GP. Be kind to yourself and recognise that the psychological and emotional symptoms are equally as challenging as the physical ones. However, these too will pass. Above all, embrace and welcome with open arms your emerging self and doing what we as women are designed to do, namely to give birth in this instance to our hag (holy one) or crone (wise one).

Libido and Relationships

'The older you get, the more you realise you have no desire for drama, conflict and any kind of intensity. You just want a cozy home, a nice book and a person who knows how you drink your coffee.'

– Anna LeMind

The research findings of a recent study published in the U.K. suggested that women of a certain age should be given testosterone on the NHS. It suggests that it might enhance women's libido and possibly improve their energy and mood, particularly during and after the menopause.

However, the researcher, Mr Panay, consultant gynaecologist, stressed that it should not be seen as Viagra for women and he went on to say that women are more complex than men and that they do not respond to the on/off button of Viagra. A GP shared a similar comment with me and supported the fact that for women, a successful sex life begins with the quality of their relationship with their partner. It is the relationship aspect of libido that I want to explore in this chapter.

As the research suggested, the loss of libido affects a percentage of menopausal women. There are other physical causes for a loss of libido during menopause and it continues to be a rather delicate subject for most and tends to be avoided or talked about, only behind closed doors. I highly recommend the books by Dr Northrup (see the chapter in resources) who writes extensively and explicitly about menopause and women's libido as we get older.

Apart from our sex lives as we age, intimacy is an important element in our relationships at whatever age.

Connecting with our partners through physical contact ensures we maintain the bonds we established in the early part of our relationships. As many of the demands of creating a home, raising children and coping with full-time careers decline, we have the time to indulge in shared sensual pleasures.

Enjoying sensual pleasures on your own and for your own benefit are as important. Take time out for a luxurious, scented bath with candles. If you are a tactile person, wearing silky PJ's or underwear or sliding between silky sheets at night or cuddling under a soft blanket with a good book, is equally vital for our overall sense of wellbeing. Wearing your favourite and signature perfume throughout the day is not an extravagance but contributes to making you feel confident about yourself.

Each one of us will have our own sensual experiences that make us feel pampered and good about ourselves. Don't feel guilty for indulging in these experiences. Making time for spoiling yourself is not only reserved for the young. Remember, if you look after yourself, you will be more able to offer assistance to others.

In support of the argument that relationships matter, researchers at Harvard University have conducted a longitudinal study over 75 years. It makes fascinating reading and the findings can be seen on TED in a talk given by Robert Waldinger, the current director for the on-going study. In essence, the findings of the research prove that social connections with others lead to health benefits and increase our longevity. In fact, as Robert Waldinger suggests, it is the knowledge that someone has your back and there is someone you can rely on when the chips are down.

There is a direct correlation between the warmth of our relationships with family, friends and a connection with the community and healthier and longer lives. The converse is also true. Those who either don't have those connections or whose relationships are less rewarding may contribute to dying younger and suffer more ill health. One of the many reasons is that the quality of our relationships increases our immunity as well as our general levels of health.

As women, our levels of happiness and satisfaction in our relationships are as important to our libido as our levels of hormones. As we get older, we may very well have been in a relationship with our partner for many years. The length of the relationship may lead to familiarity and comfort and possibly, complacency.

I have shared my belief with you elsewhere that the relationship we have with ourselves has a significant effect on our relationship with others. It sounds so selfish; I hear you say. We are socialised from the minute we come into this world to nurture and look after others. It is our raison d'être, the reason we are on earth. As women, we are the ones who have the babies and therefore do most of the nurturing. It is a biological fact. And, of course, to do so is a fundamental part of what makes us human. However, I also believe that we need to nurture ourselves in equal measures and would go so far as to say that it is our responsibility to do so.

Let's take the analogy of a well. Unless the well is continuously replenished with the life-giving water for others to come and draw on when needed, the well will become dry and dusty. It will, therefore, be unable to serve its purpose by sustaining those who rely on it.

Like the well, you need to replenish your own needs in order to have the strength, energy, physical, mental and emotional resources to support others. In fact, it is selfish not to. The upshot is that we need to be emotionally available to ourselves in the first instance before we can be emotionally available to others.

Accepting ourselves warts and all is a tall order for most of us. I certainly do not suggest for one minute that we need to strive for perfection, we are constantly evolving and developing, but it is being contented with where we are at any stage of our lifelong journey. Don't take this as a license for not taking others into account or not working on your rough edges. It isn't, but it is also not a license for ignoring your own needs and wants at the expense of others.

119

I wrote a book as a tribute to my gay brother and his partner and their journey with terminal cancer, entitled *Goodnight Doll*. In it, I discussed how difficult it was for them growing up and living as a gay couple and the need to constantly censor their actions and words for the purpose of hiding their true identity. It is exhausting, to say the least, to be ever on guard to edit ourselves thereby complying and conforming to the expectations of others. The danger is that we may move so far away from our centre that we may not find our way back again or have an arduous journey in doing so.

I have mentioned at various points in the book the importance of planning for retirement to include considerations other than the financial aspects of retirement. Equally important is recognising that your relationship with your significant other may very well be different from the relationship you shared during the years of pursuing careers and raising a family if you had children. Unless discussed and negotiated, these changes may result in unresolved tensions.

Even in the best of relationships, retirement can potentially challenge relationships in a way that you could not have anticipated. It may take some time to adjust to a whole new way of coexistence. It is the time when incompatibility and diverse interests become apparent without the distraction of separate careers. Necessary compromises on both sides will sometimes lead to the curtailment of the life of one of the parties.

Margo shares her story of the changes and challenges in her relationship with her husband of 44 years, which reflects the experiences of so many couples. She felt that in their 50s, there were more external demands made on them as a couple. Careers took up a lot of time and energy as did the raising of a family. Time spent together was often limited and not always harmonious. However, after retirement and into their 60s, there is a lot less 'push and pull'. Furthermore, now as an older woman, she is much more accepting of herself and requires less emotional input from her partner.

This is a familiar story. As we get older, we gain in confidence and an acceptance of who we are as a person. Margo and her husband now have time for more joint projects as opposed to pursuing individual goals often associated with busy jobs and careers. She describes their physical relationship as less about passion and desire and more about companionship and affection. The spark remains, however, and despite a marriage of some 45 years, they continue to have the energy to disagree strongly and voice their opinions with gusto!

Tracey reflects on how her relationship changed with her husband. Although she decided she did not want to retire and continued to work part-time and pursue her own endeavours. There was also less competition between her and her husband as to whose job was more important and therefore, more ownership with the domestic responsibilities. They have given each other the space to pursue hobbies and interests independently. The result is they now enjoy their time and pursuits together in a collegiate way as friends and partners, not as competitors.

Men and women adjust differently to retirement and much of this is based on gender roles and identity, which determines the quality of retirement. In most cases, men have had stronger occupational attachments than women who have had more non-work-related networks. Men in particular struggle with the loss of status and identity provided by their careers. These changes may very well manifest itself in the domestic sphere and the sharing of domestic duties.

Planning for retirement should include discussions around negotiating the division of domestic duties. If not, women may find that retirement has brought no respite from responsibilities and if anything, increased the time they are 'on duty' due to additional demands and expectations of a partner that is at home most of the time. Equally, it may be difficult for women to relinquish some of the domestic activities having had predominant responsibility for the home before retirement.

Retirement may very well enhance the quality of the relationship between couples or have a detrimental influence especially when there are differences in expectations of roles. As women are younger than men in general, they may want to continue with their careers after the retirement of their partners. Unless the man has planned on how he wants to spend his time after retirement, he may become resentful at being at home alone and having a partner who wants time for herself to relax after a busy day.

Advice is that couples absolutely need to have activities and interests they can share, but of equal importance is independence and time to devote to their own interests and hobbies. An increasing trend in later life is for couples when entering new relationships after divorce or loss of a partner, to keep their independence and live apart. It may be that older couples attach different values to relationships after the need for family formation has passed.

In conclusion, my reflections are that we have many relationships with many different facets to each of them. However, all our relationships flow from the relationship we, first of all, have with ourselves.

Positive Ageing

'Ageing is an extraordinary process where you become the person you always should have been.'

– David Bowie

We must be ever vigilant of the subtle and explicit narratives in relation to ageing that surrounds every aspect of our lives. Our responsibility is not to collude with these negative narratives that will worm their way into our subconscious and erode our confidence and sense of physical and emotional wellbeing. Guard against stereotypes that brainwash us to believe that ageing is not something to look forward to. It erroneously suggests that we will end up depressed, lonely, dependent, comically incapable of using smartphones and other technical devices and will become prone to bore everyone around the dinner table with out-dated stories.

The Japanese have a wise saying, namely, 'wabi-sabi', which suggests that imperfections, age, brokenness and general run-down appearance are actually considered beautiful. Not only does it refer to the human condition, but also furniture and objects with dents, scratches and layers of fading paint. It may very well be the inspiration for our Western love and appreciation of shabby chic and the willingness to pay handsomely for such items. So, instead of trying to hide your imperfections, take comfort that you too will be beautifully shabby chic. There is indeed beauty in imperfection.

The first step towards ageing positively is to be mindful of the choices we make. The most important choice that will determine our wellbeing is whether to be miserable and defeatist about the passing sands or to choose an upbeat and positive habit. Whichever one we choose will create our reality. The language we use to describe our state of mind and how we view the journey of ageing is a powerful indication as to the self-fulfilling prophecies we are creating. Whichever mindset we choose to adopt will in time become a habit. So, choose wisely.

Positive ageing is so much more than merely a philosophical concept. It is a practical way of living that we choose every day from the moment we open our eyes until we close them again at night. It is the recognition that our mind is powerful in determining the quality, or not, of our day-to-day lives and experiences. It is not a Pollyanna delusion that if we merely chant a positive mantra, everything will be hunky-dory. Instead, it is a conscious recognition of the power of the mind over our experiences of life and the reactions to that which crosses our path; both positive and negative.

I am somewhat uncomfortable with the adjective 'successful', which raises the question for me as to how do we define such success? What would we expect to see? How does 'unsuccessful' compare and who decides the criteria by which we will determine 'success' or 'failure'? What makes them the experts to define 'successful' or 'unsuccessful' on behalf of the rest of us?

The word 'success' implies that those who do not meet its definition are unsuccessful or will be deemed a failure. In defence of the ageing successful movement, it attributes its motivation in an effort to move beyond the 'decline and loss' paradigm. The study of successful ageing has grown in popularity and has become an important psychological approach contributing to the development of social theory associated with ageing. At least, the rhetoric is not about being anti-ageing.

I made reference to a Pollyanna approach elsewhere, which in its extreme denies reality. It is a fact that I find physical exertion more of a challenge. However, I continue to enjoy daily yoga and can walk a number of miles at a time. What I am losing in physical agility, I am making up with the confidence gained through the integration of the knowledge and skills I've accumulated over the years.

I have also grown to like myself and am very comfortable in my own skin. I have ditched the need to please everyone and feel guilty when I can't meet the expectations of others. This is a mantra most women have shared with me. Vanessa concurs and said that she has reached a welcome calmness without being subjected to feelings of anxiety and the need to conform to the expectations of others.

I now have the time and capacity to stop and enjoy the seasons, relishing small things and just enjoy the moment. I savour the gift of calmness that ageing has brought. The anti-ageing rhetoric means many older people feel unnecessary guilty, ashamed and useless. Feeding and accepting this negative story leads to a self-fulfilling prophecy, reducing life expectancy and quality of life.

One disease that frightens most of us as we age is that of dementia and again, the media focus on sensationalising the damage it causes to both the sufferer as well as the family. I am not denying or rejecting the real distress people experience with dementia, nor the challenges their loved ones face as a result. We have a family member who showed early onset of dementia at a fairly young age and has been very sad and distressing to witness his decline and the upheaval and pain caused to the immediate family.

However, we need to put the facts of dementia and any other aspect of ageing into context, detaching it from emotive media coverage. Research is proving that major diseases including dementia, is on the decline. It is not only attributed to the improved medical treatments we have had the benefit of in recent years, but also the changes in lifestyle choices we are making. Our diets are much healthier, smoking has become socially unacceptable, we are much more active at all ages and above all, we have a much healthier and positive attitude to ageing.

This again proves that so much of the quality of our lives is within our own sphere of influence, negating the need to feel guilty about getting older. In fact, the baby boomer generation has been observed to have better health and is more physically active than preceding generations, therefore, resulting in less cost to society. Research also suggests that approximately a quarter of our health bills are spent in the last year of our life and does not increase with age as popular belief would suggest.

I have discussed at length the assumptions surrounding the so-called cost of ageing to society. It is worth revising the guilt associated with the cost of social care. However, it is the older generation who tends to become much more involved in voluntary services for obvious reasons. The benefit to society is that the older generation contributes significantly to the reduction of government expenditure on welfare. Many of you are part of the sandwich generation managing busy careers, supporting growing teenage children and on top of all of this, being the main carer for ageing parents.

Of course, there are downsides to getting older as there is with every age. Each stage of life has its benefits as well as its drawbacks. So, why should the second half of life be any different? However, as with any other age in life, there are so many advantages and the more we focus on these as opposed to the negatives, the more likely we will be able to enjoy our later years and share our experiences and wisdom with the rest of society, given the opportunity.

Therefore, let us not focus on the unavoidable adverse effects of ageing and instead find the positives that go a long way in making our lives enjoyable and productive. I once again remind you of what H.A.G.S. stand for. So, many of the sources that lead to a healthy and positive experience of later life is within our control.

In fact, there is no excuse in creating positive experiences. You don't have to strive to become prime minister, president or start the next Amazon or Google. It is about changing your lifestyle, reinventing your wardrobe, eat healthier, have a new hairdo, start a daily walk, do yoga, etc., etc. Bottom line, there is nowhere to hide and age is no excuse for being lazy or giving up and becoming a slob. We can find joy, a purpose in life and be useful and relevant to society. Above all, we can be useful to ourselves by living a fulfilling life. Furthermore, we owe it to ourselves by making the most of the life we've been given.

We also owe it to the next generation to challenge the erroneous assumptions about life as we get older and to be role models of the lived experience of many older people. Margarette is a good example of a woman who after turning 50 considered it a priority to set a good example for her daughters. She wants her life to be an example to them as they are growing up and having to make difficult decisions. She wants their memories of her to inspire them to be courageous in chasing their dreams.

In her 50s, she left a secure job that had meant she could provide financially for her children during a long period as a single mum. She started a new business and went back to university to study a subject in which she was always interested. She resisted the voices in the wider family who told her it was too big a risk and that she shouldn't be foolish in following her 'madcap' dreams.

These were the same arguments she heard from them years ago at the age of 18. It was a risk, but to her, it was worth it and her daughters supported and cheered her on. She reflects on the fact that they are closer now than they have ever been because she thinks they are not afraid to talk to her now about their own dreams and fears and vulnerabilities. For her, this was one of the biggest rewards in pursuing her 'madcap' ideas.

Margarette's story is also one of resilience. I dedicate a chapter on the subject of resilience, but it is worth pointing out again that resilience is both mental as well as physical in nature. Both aspects of resilience result in a positive experience of ageing. A positive view of growing older perceives ageing as a natural and continuous development of being human and not abnormal and to be avoided or resorting to feelings of guilt.

Advice on how to experience wellbeing in our older age consistently offers the same message. The crunch is that it is influenced by our lifestyles, intellectual engagements, leisure activities and learning new skills. So, strive to be H.A.G.S. with attitude! It is never too late to start. In fact, research supports my challenge to you that age is no excuse for being lazy both physically and mentally. I agree with the mere fact that you are retired and have the time to pursue does not automatically lead to a happy life ever after. It is up to us to seek out new experiences. Find joy, a purpose in life and be useful and relevant to society and above all to ourselves.

I woke up this morning to BBC Radio 4 to hear of yet another excellent example of a woman who did not consider herself too old to pursue her goal of writing. Margaret Ford published her first book, *A Daughter's Choice*, at 93. It is based on 633 romantic letters between her and her husband, Jim. It is a story about her life, starting with her birth in 1926 in a Lancashire town. It continues with the love story she shared with her husband, Jim and the love letters he sent her, three a day to be precise, whilst serving with the Border Regiment during the World War II. The book concludes with their marriage in 1946. Jim being such a prolific writer, means she has more love letters to write a planned sequel. How is that for inspiration?

As an academic, I have worked a lot with younger people and instead of comparing myself to them and lamenting the loss of youth, I have realised how much I have to contribute to others in society, including the younger generation. One of the many valuable skills we have learnt over the years is that of emotional intelligence. It certainly is a valuable skill in my repertoire as a coach. It is difficult for the younger generation to understand that some things, such as emotional intelligence, you learn only with time and experience. Life after 50 can be just as meaningful and rewarding, if not more so as life before 50. If you stop and think about it, you have had 50 years of practice to become the best version of yourself. So, celebrate it daily!

I Could Have Danced All Night!

'We don't stop playing because we grow old. We grow old because we stop playing.'

– George Bernard Shaw

That is precisely what I did. Continuing with my year-long celebration of my swinging sixties, my husband and I booked a summer cruise in the Mediterranean. I have always loved dancing but never had a partner with whom to share my passion. My husband wanted to go to a rock bar where some music from his 60s era was being played by a live band. I watched two young children on separate occasions with fascination and envy as they burst into spontaneous dancing and enjoying the music in a way that reflected a lack of inhibition and self-consciousness.

Their joy reminded me of a quote I came across a photograph of a small girl exuberantly enjoying jumping and running around in the rain. The caption read, 'Do you remember her? She is still there hidden away somewhere.' It further reminded me of some words of wisdom I discovered during the research for my book. It suggested that it is better to act your shoe size instead of your perceived age. Our shoe size is likely to represent the curiosity, imagination, energy, playfulness and creativity we had when we were children. Of significance also for us, as we get older is the lack of concern with time.

That spurred me on to get off my chair in the club and I literally danced the night away, allowing that child with a love and zest for dancing to once again come out and lose herself in the music. Giving myself permission to do so and sharing my joy of the music and atmosphere allowed others to do the same. Most of them were women with a few around my age coming up to me and thanking me for being the brave one that gave them the courage to follow my lead.

All I can say is thank you for my daily exercise regime as I danced the youngsters under the table and got up the following morning with muscles not aching as much as I had anticipated. However, even if they did, it would have been worth it. I had a ball!

Oh, we take ourselves way too seriously. It was such a joyful experience reconnecting with the child within who loved and fearlessly sought adventures, discarding the voice of caution and not seeing the potential danger lurking in every situation. Or thinking I would look foolish dancing on my own all night.

My father always associated me with the child who rushes in where angels feared to tread and it was good to flex the devil-may-care muscle once again after many years of being 'sensible'. However, I am at the same time embracing the understanding and wisdom I have amassed over the years. It is not an either-or and both can live happily together.

I am delighted to have discovered an article in the *Sunday Times* during the time of writing that I am by no means the only one indulging in the joys of dancing. The Royal Academy of Dance launched a silver swans programme a few years ago in order to train a further 1,000 teachers. It was necessary to meet the demand of the over 55s interested in taking up ballet as a pastime. As these groups of swannabes discover dancing benefits in so many aspects of our lives, such as physical exercise, improved balance, creating new friendships and social connections and above all, higher levels of self-confidence.

It has taken me at least three years after reducing my working commitments to give myself permission to enjoy the things I had looked forward to doing but didn't have the time when in full-time employment. I can guarantee for those of you still gainfully employed that you will wonder how on earth you will fill your days. Like me, you may also have the fear of endless days, months and years stretching ahead of you not knowing how to occupy yourself.

I can also guarantee that it won't be long before you ask yourself, 'How did I have the time to work?' You will join the ranks of retirees who regularly chant the same mantra. It may take time to adjust to a new lifestyle. It certainly did to me. It may be a rare treat to do nothing for bursts of time when you are embroiled in full-time employment.

However, inactivity for long periods at a time is not an option when you retire. The G in H.A.G.S. emphasises the need to get up and go and keep moving. A system that stagnates is a system that dies and we human beings are a system that needs to move, engage with new and stimulating activities and be challenged both physically and mentally. A sedentary lifestyle leads to physical as well as mental decline. Our bodies were designed to keep moving and keep working. In fact, in societies where old age is an accepted part of life, the elderly remains vigorous and active in ways not practised elsewhere, especially in the West.

The assumed inevitable decline that will come to all of us in old age is mainly due to such erroneous expectations, followed by slowing down and ultimately a sedentary lifestyle. By choosing an intention to live an active and purposeful life, many of us can dramatically improve our abilities, physical strength and above all our mental responses. This reinforces the mind-body connection and the power our attitude and beliefs can and do exercise over our physical wellbeing. Fundamentally, therefore, challenge the saying to 'take it easy' as we get older as nothing could be further from the truth.

So many women have shared with me their determination not to slow down and watch the world go by, but instead, pursue their dreams now that they have the time. Dorothy is just one of many who is determined to live life to the full, despite being the sandwiched carer for a number of years. She wanted to keep on working and fulfil her dreams. She and her husband bought a vintage soft-top car and go adventuring whenever they can. Dorothy echoes the approach of so many women I spoke to, namely to pursue a life they wanted now that they do not have caring commitments and fulltime careers and the demands that come with it. More importantly, they all share their increased confidence and commitment to live their lives on their terms and being in charge of their destinies.

I have always enjoyed walking in nature and I am privileged to live in and around beautiful natural spots, providing idyllic walking conditions. I have always found it therapeutic to get away from my study and the computer screen for my daily walk with my doggies. However, I was always conscious of time ticking away and the need to get back to my office and whatever commitment I was working on at the time. I found it very difficult to allow myself to relax totally and just enjoy my surroundings and this feeling still lurks in the background. I have to regularly chastise myself that I can enjoy my environment without urgency or guilt. The Calvinistic work ethic raising its head again!

One of my forbidden pleasures was to take a book and while away some time at my favourite coffee shop, wrapping the sounds of chat and laughter around me like a cosy blanket. I would occasionally look up to indulge in another favourite pass time of mine, namely people watching. However, these times were few and far between as I could not justify wasting the time, as I perceived it.

Furthermore, any reading I did always related to my work and the research I was working on at the time. Reading purely for the sake of it was a luxury I only allowed myself when on holiday and then limited to one book a year only. Having fun was an unknown land. Not only did I not have the time, but it would have been very difficult for me to allow myself to indulge in what I would have perceived as frivolous activities. The work ethic my father instilled in us was very much alive and kicking in my psyche and duty came before pleasure.

I now have to start from scratch finding new authors whose books I want to read and it is truly an adventurous journey of discovery. Furthermore, I can now write in an unrestricted manner as I do not have to please pedantic reviewers nor chase the challenges of publishing in prestigious journals. However, having conformed to the constraints for so long, it is very difficult to find your own voice. This book is the result of that journey.

One of the few pleasures I allowed myself was a lie in over the weekends. It meant I could get up at around 8:00 am as opposed to 5:30 am or 6:00 am. For nearly two years, I continued with this practice, justifying it to myself by saying that if I had a lie in every day, it would no longer be a treat. I have finally come to realise that the world would not come to an end if I got up every morning at 8:00 am. However, I have since discovered how beneficial yoga is and being a natural morning person, I now choose to get up at 7:00 am. It allows me some quiet time to practice my yoga and meditation before the household gets up and we start the day.

I still enjoy the sense of wickedness when during the winter, in particular, I can turn around and snuggle down further under the duvet when I wake up early, pitying the poor workers who have to brace the cold and embark on another day of stressful commuting and waiting on a dark, wet and windy railway platforms or stuck in endless traffic jams. I remember those days well!

It will take time to get over the nagging guilt that plague you when engaged in perceived forbidden pleasures once you retire. Each one of us has to find our own strategy in achieving it. It is worth the effort, though. One thing I can guarantee is that once you start learning to relax and enjoy yourself, it becomes easier and addictive. It also has an element of truancy to it. However, there is no headmaster lurking in the shadows, ready to administer the appropriate punishment.

Another point to consider that may help develop the fun muscle is that the spillover benefits to the rest of your life from enjoying yourself and indulging in activities that give you pleasure will be enormous. This thought will help to rid yourself of the guilt for having fun. As with anything it takes practice, so start practising.

I do have a confession to make wherein one area in my life, I continue to struggle with the ability to let go of any urgency and that is when I get behind the wheel of a car. I have always loved driving any form of vehicle, but not paddling along at ten miles or more below the speed limit, as many older drivers do regularly. Why would I want to drive at 30 when the speed limit says 40 is acceptable? Maybe one day, I might extend my pleasure of just being in the moment to my driving and not get agitated if the journey takes five minutes more.

After 50, we have come full circle. When we were young, our unique selves emerged and found ways to express itself. However, as the years went by through education, socialisation and the responsibilities that dominated our lives, that same self was tucked away in the back of a drawer or cupboard. We learnt to conform with and adapt to the expectations of others and the responsibilities that come with growing up into young adults.

However, during the mature phase of our lives, it is time to get reacquainted with the facets of ourselves that may have remained hidden for a very long time. This is our time. Having done all the productive and duty things, it is time for us. Brush off the cobwebs and layers of accumulated dust that have hidden your dreams for so many years. But who are you? What are those dreams? Can you even remember? Be a H.A.G. with attitude and rediscover your identity!

If you have already retired or reduced your working hours as I have done, you may also have enjoyed the luxury of indulging in what brings you joy. Having conformed to the constraints and expectations of an institution during the many years of employment, I initially found myself floundering when these constraints were no longer part of my life. I struggled to decide how to divide my time between the many activities I wanted to pursue, not to mention managing the feelings of guilt in doing so.

Although I have developed a portfolio career that includes a number of activities, I no longer have the demands of a full-time academic career. I continue to devote a proportion of my time to my passion for working with others on a one-to-one basis as a coach as well as some academic-related activities.

However, it does mean I have more leisure time and above all a control over how I want to spend that time.

It is finally time when I can once again satisfy my yearning for creativity. Other than my foray into fashion designing at the beginning of my career, I have not had the opportunity to express and explore my love of design and colour. However, now is the time to rekindle my love for creativity. For the last few weeks, I have wallowed in the sheer joy of playing with colours and fabrics whilst decorating my house. I also rediscovered the purpose of my sewing machine and indulged in the joy of making my own curtains.

It was bliss to enjoy these activities without rushing and managing the time constraints of fitting it into holiday time or over the odd weekend. I have also discovered the joy of restoring and painting old furniture, giving them a new lease on life. A whole new area of creativity has been opened to me. Furthermore, as most of the pieces of furniture come from charity shops, I am also able to make a contribution to valuable causes.

As an academic, my life has centred around books, computers and lecture theatres and the pleasure of having the time to explore nature has been one of the rewards of having more leisure time. This week I have relished the arrival of the first spring flowers.

My own experiences of the last few weeks have once again reminded me that there are so many different forms of creativity. It is not restricted to painting pictures or drawing. There is a creativity to suit everyone and taking the time to discover what yours might be is worth the effort.

Quality vs Quantity

'Things of quality have no fear of time.'

– Todd Herschberg

An advertisement for slow holidays on a national radio station recently reminded me of the slow movement I came across in the late 90s. In essence, it is a cultural revolution against the idea that faster is always better. Instead, it is about seeking to do everything at the right speed.

The slow movement has gained momentum since it was established in the 80s in Italy and its first association with food. It reflected the fear of globalisation and the impact on farming and traditions with food. Its purpose was to defend and protect regional traditions and a slower pace of life. In particular, the unique Mediterranean tradition of time spent with family and friends over gastronomic pleasures washed down with local wines.

The slow movement can now be found in areas such as fashion, design and even journalism. In Britain, the BBC recently experimented with slow TV and featured a two-hour canal boat journey down the Kennet and Avon Canal. The journey was without commentary or music and with only the sounds of the countryside and the lapping of the water to accompany the visual aspect of the journey; very relaxing and calming.

It is, however, a concept we find very difficult and the word 'slow' tends to be associated with being lazy and someone who doesn't pull their weight. Many cultures, the west, in particular, value speed and producing as much as we possibly can in less time. We have come to value quantity over quality. We also associate success with busyness, but often it leads to burnout. In our Western societies with its drive to achieve, strive and win, there is significant wisdom in the harmony of moving gently and with an open mind to the needs of the moment, being in tune with the pace and flow of the unfolding day.

The stress and pressures of daily life resonate with advice from research which suggests that our lifestyle choices are even more important than our genes when it comes to ageing. Although we can't discount the genes and their influence on our health and wellbeing, the lifestyle choices we make will determine whether the bad genes become active and pose a serious threat to our health in later life.

It is the latter that the slow movement questions and challenges us to shift our focus for the benefit of quality over quantity in everything we do, including how we live. The purpose is to structure our lives around meaning and fulfilment. In other words, the quality of our life. We have lost the art of doing nothing and merely just being rather than cram every second of the day with some form of doing.

The movement advocates connection, a connection to life and above all a connection to ourselves and the natural rhythms that guide our lives. To achieve connection requires us to slow down our mind in order to see what we need for the wellbeing of ourselves and others. Not only are there external rhythms that guide our daily activity such as the rising of the sun, the changes of the seasons but also internal rhythms.

We have lost touch with these various rhythms in both nature and within ourself to our own detriment. We have tried to speed up the natural flow of things for the profit at our own cost. The way we produce our food is just one such example. Women, in particular, are affected by daily and monthly cycles that guide our energy, moods and sleep. When our lives are in sync with these rhythms, life flows a lot more easily, resulting in heightened satisfaction with life.

Each one of us has our own rhythm as well as the different rhythms of the stages of our lives. The slow movement advocates developing awareness and connection to these rhythms and cycles to enhance the quality of our lives. This whole concept becomes a reality when we either fully retire or reduce our hours at work. It is also the perfect time to reflect on how the philosophies of the movement can assist us in creating a rewarding phase in our lives.

The challenge is in allowing ourselves to slow down and consciously make an effort to change our approach to life. From personal experience, it potentially takes a long time in achieving this idyllic state. However, the sooner we start, the sooner we will be prepared for a rich and rewarding new phase in our lives when we eventually reduce our time in employment.

Slowing down is not about giving up or becoming a couch potato. It's about allowing life and new experiences to come knocking at our door and being able to hear the knock. The need to keep active and exercise as we get older does not mean frantically rushing around and feeling guilty. Instead, it is about savouring the pleasure of just being and enjoying the moment, whatever that might be for you.

In doing so, we will be able to recognise the many benefits of getting older. Slowing down as we get older allows us to deepen our experiences and become more aware of the simple pleasures in life. Furthermore, in practising slowing down it allows us to enjoy everyday events which may have passed us by in busy lives when we were younger. We now have the time to witness the changes in nature around us, savour the many subtle flavours in our food, enjoying calm and inspiring music.

My advice and suggestion are to start daily with a few minutes to just being. Instead of having a coffee or a sandwich while working, take those few moments to connect to the taste and the quality of the food and simply to enjoy what you are eating or drinking. You would be surprised how many subtle flavours and textures you discover in what you eat and drink. Rather than check emails or planning your next activity when finding yourself in a queue, take the time to consciously observe your environment and the people around you. Above all, take time to truly connect and be present when engaging with your loved ones, instead of having one eye on your smartphone or tablet.

I mentioned above that even the fast pace industry of fashion is open to the slow movement. Being of a certain age we know that fashion comes and goes. In fact, the official verdict is that fashion is dead. However, style lives on and is very personal. If we keep hearing the same thing, albeit, in slightly different ways, there has to be some an element of truth in it.

Reflecting the philosophies of the slow movement is that of the Danish hygge, pronounced hooga, approach to life that popped up everywhere in the media at the time of writing. But what exactly is it? It is always a challenge to translate words from one language to another. Words convey the meaning that could vary significantly from one language and culture to another.

The Danish concept of hygge is one such example. In essence, it is about cosiness and togetherness, feeling safe and contented. As the Danes are rated as one of the happiest people in the world, there has to be something worth exploring in the concept of living the hygge way.

Different cultures have words that say more or less the same thing. The Danish word hygge comes from a Norwegian word meaning wellbeing. The German equivalent is *gemütlichkeit* and the Dutch call it *gezelligheid*, broadly speaking, conveying the same meaning. The English translation is loosely referred to as cosiness, but needless to say, there is a lot more to it than that. It is, in fact, a way of life. It reminds me of the French concept of joie de vivre.

Hygge does not merely represent a way of living during the winter, but something the Danes practice throughout the year. However, with 17 hours a day of darkness in the depths of winter, it helps to cope with the long, cold winters. Whereas the summer hygge way of life includes activities such as picnics and barbecues, outdoor concerts and festivals, other activities to commune with nature such as bicycle riding, walking and many other outdoor pursuits.

The theme which is repeated throughout all the discussions and definitions of the term hygge is about creating a warm and inviting atmosphere to share with family and friends. Picture sitting in front of a crackling fire on a cold winter's night, wrapped up in a woolly jumper, sipping mulled wine, hot chocolate, coffee or whatever tipple takes your fancy and you will begin to get a sense of what the word encompasses.

It is associated with family and friends getting together to share a meal, while away the time exchanging ideas and talking about what matters in life, often accompanied by candlelight. Candles clearly play a significant role in living the hygge way as the Danes are one of the biggest consumers of candles in the world.

However, it is also time spent on one's own engaged in activities that give one a sense of wellbeing whatever that might be. It reflects the notion of being kind to oneself. It is certainly not about extravagance but more about indulgence in the small, pleasurable things of life as opposed to the expensive next having to own gadget, which becomes obsolete after a few months.

The philosophy of the slow movement reflects loosely the concept of hygge and encourages us to slow down the pace of our very hectic lives. Instead, it advocates not focusing on doing things faster but to do things better. The emphasis is on the quality over quantity in everything we do. From a mindfulness perspective, it is also about being present in the moment, savouring the activity we are engaged in rather than racing ahead at speed to the next one.

Whatever word you wish to use, for me, it is about cherishing oneself and appreciating the small pleasures of life that provide us with a sense of well-being and contentment. It also reflects the joy and pleasure we receive when we connect with others in our social circle, whether friends or family. It is once again a reminder of the research that has proved beyond doubt that social connections are important for our overall wellbeing and longevity.

We have looked towards science and the medical profession for cures associated with ageing such as cancer, heart disease, Alzheimer's and dementia to name a few. However, we fail to appreciate that a significant percentage of healthy ageing rests with us and the choices we make on a daily basis. Medicine is not the only solution and much of our physical and mental health are the results of the life choices we make.

Throughout the book, I make reference to our attitude and the lifestyle choices that have a significant impact on the quality of our lives. Not only what we eat and whether we take the time to exercise or not, but the quality of our thoughts, feelings and assumptions. I love the way Deepak Chopra phrased it, 'Our cells are constantly eavesdropping on our thoughts and being changed by them.'

It reinforces research that suggests the choices we make, including our mental activities, have a significant impact on the quality of our lives. The concept of hygge and that of the slow movement clearly recognises that leading a joyful and fulfilling life helps to maintain our health and in so doing, extend our lives.

Ignoring the commercialisation of the concept, I once again encourage you to take the time to look after yourself so that you will be able to look after others. Replenish your well so that there will be enough to share with others.

A slower lifestyle will also allow us to collect valuable and meaningful memories to treasure vs racing ever onwards to the next deadline or goal. Adding variety and novelty to our lives will enhance and enrich those memories. The challenge is therefore to be in tune with life and willing to engage with new and novel experiences and avoid the repetition and comfort of routine.

Not only will novelty add to a richer and more colourful life, but it will also keep our minds active and stimulated. It will also make us more interesting to be with rather than regurgitating the same stories and experiences, which our families and friends would know off by heart.

Technology for Oldies

'Once we accept our limits, we go beyond them.'
                                                    – Albert Einstein

It is a statistical fact that year on year the ageing population is growing. However, all our lives are becoming more intimately intertwined with technology irrespective of age. Yet technology continues to be designed by younger people for the young. However, very soon, one in five consumers will be in their later life and companies ignore this group at their peril. It is just another example of the older generation becoming invisible.

It would be imminently sensible for companies at the forefront of designing new technology to include in their research and development an awareness of why and how older adults choose to use their devices. Our needs differ greatly from those of the younger generation. Another interesting fact is that the use of tablets is far higher among the 65-year-olds than the national average in the U.K. If that is the case, how, if at all, is the technology adapted to take this into account?

There are some differences between us oldies and the younger generation when it comes to our needs of technology. In the first instance, our vision tends to diminish, as we get older. In order for websites and apps to be attractive to the older generation, they need to give consideration to size and font size, allowing users to adjust these to meet their particular individual requirements. Some software providers already offer this option.

Apart from the physical design of technology, of equal importance is the psychological aspect of its use. Designers of products need to understand the relationship older users have with technology, including their concerns about the use of modern technology. Not addressing these issues may very well alienate potential users from their products. One such example is the very real concern regarding the safety and security of our personal identities.

One of the cardinal sins committed by designers is the making of assumptions. These assumptions tend to be associated with a much younger generation and their knowledge, experience and expectations of technology and its use. People who haven't grown up with computers and smart devices interact very differently with technology.

One example of the difference between the generations is that of managing short-term memory loss. This will vary from individual to individual, but the older we get, the more we rely on the use of calendars and diaries to support our memories. Technology has tremendous potential in this one area alone to provide timely and paperless reminders of important actions. I couldn't survive without the electronic reminders to ensure I turn up at meetings at the appropriate time, not forgetting important appointments through to staying up to date with the to-do list.

An interesting fact that designers may not necessarily be aware of is that the older generation excels when it comes to attention span, persistence and thoroughness. This is particularly significant when the average person's attention span has dropped to below that of a goldfish. The relevance is that older people will notice things that younger people may skip over. On the flip side, the pace of completing a task will be slower.

The benefits of modern technology to the older generation, especially if they have mobility problems, are endless. Furthermore, it has the power to support individuals in staying connected with the world in the comfort of their own homes. A possible problem for many older people is issues of social isolation resulting in feelings of loneliness. Various forms of social media and methods of staying in touch with friends and family offer a lifeline to homebound people.

Technology that takes into account the differing needs of an older generation can single-handedly make a monumental contribution to supporting people to remain independent. Not only does the design of technology with older people in mind make business sense, but it also makes moral sense. As the older generation, we have a responsibility to engage with technology for our own benefit. Embracing its benefits will continue to support our independence and put us in charge of our own lives. There is very little that cannot be achieved via technology from the comfort of our own homes.

Most, if not all, retail companies offer an online facility to order anything from your weekly shop all the way through to sophisticated financial transactions and everything in between. It has been my desire to integrate regular yoga practice into my life for some years but given the demands of my travelling schedule, this has been virtually impossible. That was until I was advised by a yoga teacher to go onto YouTube and access yoga classes online. It has made a significant difference to my life and now wherever I may find myself, my online yoga teacher, Yoga with Adrienne, is ready and waiting to put me through my paces.

There really is no excuse for engaging in activities via technology that will enhance our lives with minimal effort. All we have to do is overcome a fear of technology if it hasn't played a part in our lives hitherto. I remind you once again of the A in H.A.G.S. and encourage you to take stock of your attitude towards technology if it is placing a barrier between you and your independence and the benefits technology can offer.

In previous chapters, I've made reference to the significant benefits associated with learning new skills as we get older. Not only does technology offer us the opportunity of independence at any age, but it also provides us with the chance for learning and thereby exercising our mental abilities. For some time now, I have used technology to support me in learning new languages. Not only does this activity go a long way in keeping my mind active, but it also has the added benefit of making my time spent in those cultures which are much more rewarding. Apart from all the obvious benefits, engaging in learning activities and managing our affairs significantly build on our self-confidence, creating positive self-fulfilling prophecies.

I cast my mind back with sadness to my mother-in-law who lost her husband in her 80s. During the many years, they were together, my father-in-law, like so many men of his generation, took care of all aspects of their affairs including the finances such as banking. She had been sheltered from all such decisions and when the time came to withdraw cash, she was unaware of cash machines and how to operate them.

It is a big leap in your 80s to go from no exposure to technology to having to navigate modern life and the benefits offered by technology. My advice is, therefore, to start now in gaining knowledge of the support it can offer. If there are no children or grandchildren around to show you the ropes, there will be a plethora of short courses offered by colleges in your area to provide you with the necessary skills and confidence.

As I mentioned earlier, it is a statistical fact that year on year, the ageing population is growing. As our lives become more intimately intertwined with technology, is it, therefore, wise that technology continues to be designed by younger people for younger people? One example of a website that has spotted the needs and interests of the older generation and responded to it is Silversurfers. Worth having a look. It is packed with both entertaining as well as informative articles and guides.

My advice to designers, therefore, is to go out and talk to your customers, both young and old. You may very well come away with product design ideas that you could never have envisaged otherwise.

I made reference above to the very legitimate fears associated with technology. Those age 75 and older are the most vulnerable when it comes to the fraud of all kinds, despite being tech-savvy. The scams range from internet, email, telephone and above else face-to-face scams. Fraud aimed at anyone no matter what their age is only likely to escalate, given that our lives are increasingly led or supported by online services.

Fraudsters, deliberately and without remorse, go out to deceive their victims with the promise of investments, goods, prizes and other fictitious pledges. Yours truly despite priding myself on my technical savvy fell foul to such a scam. Luckily, it did not result in a loss of savings, but the whole experience was scary and upsetting, to say the least. Another critical reason why we need to educate ourselves is the benefits and pitfalls of technology.

In my opinion, the worse of those ruthless fraudsters are the ones who have the gall to rob people face-to-face of their savings on the threat of fraudulent home and emergency repairs. There was a spate of such daylight robbery in my area by a group of cowboy builders recently. Fortunately, they were caught and brought to justice, but it will not necessarily lead to compensation for their victims for the loss of savings or the trauma caused by the whole experience. It made me think as to why the older generation is more likely to be victims of fraud.

Whatever the fraud, there are common elements to be found in most frauds. In the first instance, the fraudsters are charismatic and gain the trust of their victims. Their actions appear to be motivated by a concern for the wellbeing of their victims or that they have deliberately been chosen or seen as lucky to be selected for whatever benefits for which they are the bearer.

Fraudsters tend to target people who are vulnerable such as those who live on their own, are at home during the day, have savings and investments and sadly, those who are lonely and therefore more likely to talk to strangers. I would add that the older generation was also brought up with values that are more insistent on being polite and not wanting to be perceived as rude and automatically extend trust towards others, including strangers. They may also be more vulnerable to intimidation and scare tactics.

Sadly, women are twice as likely to be the victim of financial scams than men. This is potentially because women in a particular age group were not used to being responsible for financial decisions, my mother-in-law being a good example. There are a number of ways in which we can protect our relatives and ourselves. Prevention is better than cure and the best way to avoid being scammed is to learn to spot the signs in advance. The following is a useful checklist to bear in mind when approached by strangers in person or online.

Being contacted without invitation. Whatever services you may be looking for from bank accounts, investments to traders, you should be the one to initiate contact. If you are contacted out of the blue, it is likely to be a pushy salesperson or worse, an attempted scam. Put the phone down immediately and if they approach you in person, don't answer your doorbell if you are not expecting visitors. Having being caught by cold callers, I have now installed a camera that sends an alert to my phone should anyone ring my doorbell. It gives me the opportunity to ignore the caller if I am not expecting anyone or if it is someone I don't know. They will eventually give up and go away.

It sounds too good to be true. If the deal, product or service sounds too good to be true, you can bet it probably is. Very few of us have relatives we've never heard of before leaving us thousands in their wills.

You are asked for personal details. Scammers are extremely skilled at getting you to reveal personal details. Should they succeed, it will give them access to your bank accounts, set up new accounts in your name or even steal your identity. The golden rule is never to reveal any personal information.

Pressure is put on you to make a decision right away. Scammers know that the more time you have to think about a decision, the more likely you will spot a scam or change your mind. Be wary of anyone who puts pressure on you to make a decision.

Emails or letters full of grammatical and spelling mistakes. Legitimate correspondence from equally legitimate companies will not be peppered with glaring mistakes.

Suspicious contact details. Understandably, scammers would be reluctant to provide you with contact details allowing them to be traced. Be suspicious, therefore, if the person tries to avoid giving contact details or provide you with a post office box number.

Alas, this is just the tip of the iceberg and scammers continue to invent more and more sophisticated and convincing ways to ensnare us in their web of deceit. Be on the alert and if in doubt, report your suspicions.

A final word on the use of technology. Don't let the fear of being scammed deny you the many benefits of using technology. Embrace it and take precautions to protect yourself and your assets. If you do not have family members around to support you in doing this, there is significant help and advice out there. Start with the supplier of your device who will guide you in setting up various protection mechanisms.

Thanks for the Memories

'My face carries all my memories. Why would I erase them?'
— Diane von Furstenberg

The practice of telling stories is as old as mankind itself. Sharing our memories and history through the telling of stories is ingrained in our psyche. It remains the way in which some cultures around the world capture and record the history of their communities.

The importance of sharing collective memory is as relevant to families as it is to communities. In the first instance, the narrator benefits significantly from sharing their stories. Our stories are among the richest resources we have for living a rich and fulfilling life. They can once again transport us to events and experiences that gave us joy and contentment. As we get older, it is vital to capture and pass on our memories to the next generation. This was brought home to me recently by a Dutch friend of mine, now in his early 90s.

He was brought up in Indonesia when it was part of the Dutch East Indies. It meant that during World War II, he and all members of his family were captured and imprisoned in the Japanese war camps for a number of years. His story is particularly poignant and offers some valuable lessons to future generations.

His memories will provide his descendants with their family history generating a sense of belonging and securing the family roots. Furthermore, they may also go some way to act as a reminder of the horrors of war not only to his own grand and great-grandchildren but also to the younger generation in general.

Documenting our memories is not only for the benefit of the generations to come but it is also of benefit to ourselves. Reminiscing is one of life's unpredictable but thrilling delights. There is a childlike pleasure associated with coming across forgotten storage boxes that contain memories of past experiences and events. These memories are testimony to the life we've led, our hopes and dreams and how far we have come as an individual.

There is an added benefit to the sharing of our memories, especially as we get older. Sharing memories helps to 'scaffold' or support our memories as we age. Research suggests that by remembering and sharing memories with our partners or family members, we are able to recall past events in greater detail. Investing time in sharing and remembering our stories, therefore, results in a cognitive benefit as well as deepening our relationships with our families.

A further benefit of writing your own life story reminds us of how much we have lived and experienced. It also highlights the positive experiences and blessings we have enjoyed throughout our lives. Writing our stories also makes us realise how much we are connected to others. Sharing your story may not only benefit your own immediate family but may offer comfort and inspiration to a much wider audience. For example, writing a blog is a great way to connect with others and to share experiences and inspiration. Sadly, we dismiss our lives and experiences as being insignificant and of no interest to others. Not true.

Not sharing our memories and experiences runs the risk of our grandchildren never really knowing who we were and what we were about; what made us sad, what brought us joy, what we're our disappointments and achievements. By not reminiscing and recording our memories, we may very well leave a traceless presence behind.

My father was such an example. His father deserted him and his mother when he was two years old. His mother subsequently remarried and his stepfather was the father from hell. The result was that he dismissed his childhood and relatives and refused to share any stories of his family. I, therefore, have almost no knowledge of his, and therefore my, relatives and ancestors.

What is perhaps less known is that memory is highly elastic. This means that we are more in control of our memories than we think and what we carry with us in terms of our personal history. Our memories have the capacity to inspire and create a sense of optimism by choosing to amplify the positive rather than merely focusing on the negative.

Photographs and artefacts are a great way to jog our memories and capture the essence of events in the past. Surrounding ourselves with precious reminders of positive experiences or people we have loved continues to enrich our lives long after events or the passing on of loved ones. I add a footnote to this and suggest a healthy attitude to artefacts from the past. They could equally lock us into our histories and deny us the joy of new experiences and adventures. Another example of attitude and the power of choosing a positive over negative filter through which to view past, present and future.

I have inherited the dining room suite that belonged to my maternal grandparents. As my mother never thought it relevant or important to share stories of what that suite meant to her parents, I have very little knowledge of their daily family life. I was borne after the death of my maternal grandmother and I was very young when my grandfather died.

However, I have many family memories of the meals, chats, debates and yes, tears shed around that table. So, I will leave my memories and stories of what our family experienced around it for the future owners to enjoy and perhaps weave into their own stories and memories they will make around the table. Memories can be lonely and therefore need to be shared. Sharing our stories with others also serves to maintain our individual and shared identities.

I know, writing our memoirs and sharing our stories is one of those things we plan to do yet keep putting off. We no doubt think 'I'll do it tomorrow'. However, remember tomorrow is now. In January 2016, I published a tribute to my gay brother and his partner and their journey with terminal cancer, entitled *Goodnight Doll*.

My motivation was to share with others their love story and dedication to each other through the good and the bad days. However, their story has made me aware of a much bigger issue that affects so many people around the world and will increase dramatically in the years to come.

The people around us preserve our stories about who we are, whom we have loved and lost, our successes and failures. We automatically assume these people include our children and grandchildren as well as our friends and family. However, there are many people ageing without children who are acutely aware of such a loss of legacy.

This was another motivating factor in publishing my tribute to my brother and his partner, namely to preserve their legacy. It is not only the LGBT community who has known the reality of being childless in a family-oriented community but also the increasing number of baby boomers, in particular, who are ageing without children.

There is another serious aspect of the LGBT community we don't consider such as the options for older couples or single people who are considering alternative living offered by retirement or assisted living residences. It is rare that such alternatives are open to non-heterosexual couples. A fact that needs to be raised and challenged. My brother and his generation of gay people spent much of their time and energy protecting themselves from the homophobia, which is still to be found in society including alternative living communities.

The political rhetoric during the last U.K. election campaign and the spotlight on social care made reference to 'older people and their families', 'selling the family home', 'older people and their relatives' and 'families must do more'. The assumption being that everyone will age surrounded by a family. Who are these 'hard-working families' who will shore up the crisis in social care? If you are not part of such a family, who will fight your corner on your behalf?

Various statistics predict that by 2030, 2 million people over the age of 65 will be without children in the U.K. I am sure other countries will be experiencing similar issues. Despite the significant demographic shift it has largely been ignored in debates on ageing. As with any complex issue, there are many factors that contribute to this but this is not a reason to sweep it under the carpet in the hope it will go away.

Being childless remains a taboo subject in many cultures. As a woman, you have not fulfilled your duty if you have not produced any offspring whether that was by conscious choice or not. Childless men around children are labelled as a suspect. An adult without children in most societies means you live on the margins of what is considered 'normal'.

However, having children is certainly no guarantee of social support in old age. My mother is testimony to this having lost both her sons and one of her daughters (me) living on the other side of the world. It is also true that in some cultures, the reason people have children is to have an insurance policy for their old age.

Society at large does not value older people who are seen as a burden and a drain on society. The abuse of older people in hospitals and care homes are regularly featured in the media. The assumption of society and politicians, as highlighted by the last U.K. election campaign, is that children will fill the gap of social care for the elderly. The unspoken expectation is that children will pick up the slack. But what if you don't have children? Who picks up the slack then?

The charity, Ageing Without Children, suggests that the fears of many people ageing without children are justified. The fear that there will not be anyone to speak up for them or that they will be ignored or mistreated in a home or by the system is real and valid. They continue to be an invisible group ignored by society and policymakers alike.

It is a reality for many people that their friends are equally ageing and in need of the same support. Furthermore, families have become much smaller and many elderly people are likely to find themselves without any immediate family or family living too far away to offer any form of care or assistance. My personal experiences bear this out having left the family home to travel and work abroad many years earlier.

As an incurable optimist, I suggest the best we can do is to put steps into place to support us in our old age whilst we can, irrespective of our personal circumstances. Then get on with living and making the most of each day and the blessings they offer.

The Secrets of Health
and Well-Being

'To thrive in life you need three bones. A wishbone, a backbone and a funny bone.'

– Reba McEntire

We have been brainwashed to believe the popular press who has associated ageing with reduced faculties, sagging skin, not to mention decaying bodies. Frankly, ageing is seen as a disease that needs to be cured. However, what is the flipside of ageing and are we told the whole truth? As I have mentioned on numerous occasions throughout the book that the secret of ageing, well, is in many instances down to the lifestyle choices more so than our genes alone.

Unless you've lived on an island for the last 20 years or so, you will know how important lifestyle is to longevity. The choices we make on many levels manifest in the quality of our health and sense of well-being.

There is enough research out there supporting the unequivocal fact that a lack of exercise is detrimental to both our physical as well as our mental health.

The G in H.A.G.S. is a reminder to get up and get going. We slow down as we get older not because of body parts ceasing up, but because we stop exercising and doing what our bodies were designed for, namely to work and keep moving physically. Being physically active may make the difference between dependence and independence.

As I mentioned in an earlier chapter, pursuing vigorous exercise and spending endless hours in a noisy, sweaty gym, is not necessarily the answer. In fact, Vanessa was advised to give up her gym membership as it was doing her arthritic knees more harm than good. Instead, regular brisk walks in nature are not only good for your body but equally beneficial to your mental wellbeing. There is nothing more rewarding than being out in nature and enjoying the ever-changing palette of the different seasons. The added bonus is that it is free and does not require expensive membership.

Indeed, there are those who, due to ill health, find it very difficult, if not impossible to exercise. You may recall from the chapter on technology that I mention the plethora of YouTube videos available on yoga and other physical pursuits, catering for all abilities. My husband has a chronic health condition and finds it very difficult to walk. However, there are many forms of exercise that can be done sitting in a chair and equally as beneficial to the body.

Many of us who have spent years hunched over computers or chained to a desk may find it a challenge to get up and go. As with everything, starting small with little but regular exercise and building up over time is the best way to proceed. A sedentary lifestyle may lead to negative changes in our personality and our ability to deal with stress.

It is understandable that being less active will significantly affect how we lead our lives and ultimately the quality of life. If we get out and about less often, we may have less opportunity for socialising and the stimulus provided by interaction with others. A downward spiral ensues. On the other hand, apart from the physical benefits exercise also has positive mood-enhancing effects.

At the time of writing, the media highlighted the danger of reaching for painkillers as a way of dealing with chronic pain that often prevents us from engaging in physical movement. The report went on to highlight how often the medical profession prescribes strong painkillers as a matter of course rather than consider offering or recommending other ways of dealing with pain.

Contrary to the reassurances of the pharmaceutical industry that patients would not become addicted to opioid pain medication, it has been proved that such medication can be highly addictive as many have found out. A healthier lifestyle may go a long way in helping us to manage pain. Pain clinics are also managing chronic pain by offering alternative therapies. So, before reaching for the painkillers, seek advice on healthier options that may be available.

Of equal importance to our health and wellbeing is our diet. Again, there is a plethora of information available at our fingertips offering guidance to a healthier way of eating. I urge you not to confuse healthy eating with bland and boring eating. Healthy eating can be both creative and pleasing to the palette. I made reference to the website, Silversurfers, aimed at those over 50 and with every issue they offer some easy, but delicious recipes for a healthier eating regime. Not only is our physical health vital to our overall wellbeing, but of equal importance is the on-going development of our mental abilities.

We may have avoided taking action to lead a healthier life and defended our choices quoting the popular belief that suggests we are who we are due to our genes. For a long time, our genes have been seen as playing a major role in what we may experience later in life, such as disease, baldness and so forth. A reminder once again that the new study of epigenetics has shown that our mental activities can equally have a powerful impact on our genes. Together with lifestyle choices, thought patterns have the ability to turn certain genes on or off.

Contrary to popular belief, the ageing brain becomes smarter. The adage of 'use it or lose it' applies to the grey matter of our brains and by using and exercising our brains, we are able to boost our brain's connectivity. What we do or don't do with our brains changes the architecture of the brain.

After years of practice, we become much better at problem-solving with an accumulation of certain types of knowledge. Furthermore, the older brain becomes much more skilled at activating both hemispheres of the brain simultaneously, enabling us to become much more accomplished at reasoning and problem-solving as we get older. I mentioned the idea of a mental gym for the brain elsewhere and that is more or less what neuroscience advises us to do.

Sorry ladies, but age is no longer an excuse when it comes to learning. You can indeed teach old dogs new tricks! It is not the domain of the young and you can learn new things no matter what age according to neuroscience. Technology has greatly contributed to the development and findings of neuroscience and real-time brain imaging in recent years. I have shared some of the findings in detail elsewhere. I can't recommend TED talks enough as both a source of entertainment, but a font of information and knowledge from reputable practitioners and scientists sharing their wisdom. Furthermore, you can access these from the comfort of your favourite armchair.

Of course, no one science has the answer to all our questions and much of the findings of neuroscience have been overhyped and exaggerated. As human beings, we are deliciously complex and can never be reduced to the findings of any research study, no matter how revolutionary. They do, however, offer some general guidance and words of wisdom on what can enhance the quality of our lives.

Neuroscience is one such example and for the moment, we can take comfort in its findings and knowledge that getting older does not necessarily mean losing our mental capacities. As a science, it has massively enhanced our understanding of how the breath-taking marvels of the human brain work. Of equal importance is that it goes a long way in helping us understand how the brain changes with age.

As the brain learns by doing, the older brain is proven to be more effective in finding solutions. Although we lose certain abilities of the brain such a short-term loss of memory as we age, we gain the ability to use and develop other parts of the brain. It is within our power to choose activities, thoughts and an attitude that will strengthen and develop our brains into middle age and beyond.

The mental fitness of our brains is significantly dependent on how we choose to use and exercise our brains. The bottom line is that healthy eating, a positive attitude, relaxation, social connections, continuous learning and regular exercise builds long-term healthy brains.

There are a number of activities that have been proved by neuroscience to have positive effects on our brains, which also has the added benefit in preventing neurodegenerative disease. Neuroscience reveals that the age of our brains is not what is of importance, but what we do with it. Exercise such as walking and dancing has the benefit of contributing to reducing the occurrence of dementia and Alzheimer's disease by keeping the mind sharp and rewiring the neural pathways of the brain. So, dig out those dancing or walking shoes and get moving!

Other mental activities that require intense mental focus, such as learning a new language or a musical instrument also affect the neural wiring of the brain. Learning builds connections thereby assisting our cognitive abilities from problem-solving to recalling information. The bottom line is we will have a much more resilient brain to deal with degeneration. H.A.G.S., remember? Let it be your daily mantra.

It is not just our brains that get wiser as we get older, but also our blood cells. Our immune systems are bombarded by millions of dangers on a daily basis. Our blood cells develop an immune memory as it ages. The result is that it spots an old enemy such as colds a mile away, jumping into action to protect us from harm. Therefore, we are less susceptible to the common cold as we get older.

The immune system, therefore, remembers enemies encountered over the years and protect us from them should they come along later in life. For allergy sufferers, the symptoms also decline in later life. In addition, migraine sufferers can also look forward to a reduction of migraines as they age.

Although stress is a fact of life, how we deal with stress can contribute to the ageing of the brain. A brain that is constantly in fight or flight mode when dealing with stress will shrink and age faster than a brain that deals more effectively with stress. Which is why meditation and mindfulness are scientifically proven to be some of the most effective ways of protecting and developing our brains. Meditation builds up the ability of the brain to maintain a positive sense of well-being during stress thereby protecting the brain from the ageing process. The inverse is also true. If we continue to focus on negativity and respond to stressful situations in a fight or flight mode, we will contribute to the damage that is inflicted on our brains.

Stress is seen as a significant contributor in reducing our overall health and wellbeing as it produces stress hormones, which impacts our ability to fight infection. Stress combined with poor lifestyle choices is a toxic combination as it accelerates the ageing process. A healthy and resilient immune system will help us to fight illnesses and speed up the recovery process should we fall ill. Avoiding excessive stress and making good lifestyle choices all contribute to strong immune systems.

We may also reject many beauty treatments as expensive, self-indulgence but massage, facials, reflexology, manicures, pedicures all go a long way in reducing stress. It is not necessary to frequent expensive health spas if it is beyond your budget. Be creative and find other ways to get the same benefit of being pampered.

Lest we forget, with age comes an increase in self-esteem. We are much happier in our own skins later in life. It might be that the wisdom we develop helps us to appreciate the transient nature of many things we thought of as being important when we were young. We recognise that our true value and worth has little to do with how we look or what we do in the world and everything to do with who we really are at a deeper level.

We also have a greater sense of positive well-being to look forward to. Negative emotions tend to decrease with age and we are less prone to the emotional rollercoaster of our youth. Thankfully our vulnerability towards stress and worry also reduces in later life, especially if we take the healthy choices mentioned in this chapter and elsewhere. Getting older sharpens the mind to realise that we have limited time on earth. We, therefore, become better at letting go of the trivial and focus on what is truly important. In addition, we also get to make fewer mistakes.

Enjoying life is not only for the young and I urge you to explore what it is that makes you feel alive and full of the joys of spring. Once you have discovered it, go out and engage in more of it as it will support you in ageing well. Ultimately, we will all discover our own unique activities and lifestyle that works for us.

The Age of Invisibility

'Women always try to tame themselves as they get older, but the ones who look best are often a bit wilder.'

– Miuccia Prada

Legend has it that vampires do not produce a reflection in a mirror. The same could be said of us women when you reach a certain age. To all intents and purposes, we become invisible to the outside world. Guaranteed to happen the further away we move from the age of 50.

We no longer receive a second glance from a stranger on the train, in a coffee bar or any other public place. We simply cease to exist. There is no specific day, month or year when this phenomenon occurs.

When we reach the age when we become invisible, we are at best ignored and at worst we are talked to as though we are once again children who should be spoken to in a language reserved for that age group. Our own attempt at intelligent conversation is ignored.

The media conspires with this and women of a certain age are rarely featured in magazines nor are our experiences and issues discussed intelligently or otherwise. Yet the world does not consist only of young, gorgeous, stick-like models. As it happens, it is the older generation who has the disposable income and therefore the ones to be courted rather than dismissed.

It may also be that we feel invisible because we no longer consider that we look young and therefore become irrelevant. If we want to remain visible, how do we go about it? I return to my mantra that our attitude and how we feel about ourselves and our lives will go a long way in making us visible because we will act with visibility.

For inspiration, I highly recommend the book by Ari Seth Cohen, *Advanced Style*, which features how older women use clothes, accessories and makeup to communicate their own unique personalities and styles. There is no doubt that the women introduced in his book will be anything but invisible to those around them. In fact, I suggest the complete opposite.

It is important not to confuse style with fashion. We each create a personal style that communicates our individual and unique personalities, rather than slavishly following the latest fashion. However, some older women are hell-bent on conspiring with the assumption that we are invisible and not worthy of a second glance and behave accordingly. Some look as though they have walked right out of a black and white movie, devoid of all colour. No wonder, they both feel invisible and are treated as though they are! Colour has the power to not only make you feel better about yourself and your life but makes you visible as well.

Our style tells the world who we are and what we are about. It is communicated in the way we wear a particular piece of jewellery, a combination of accessories, the way we tie or drape, a scarf or the colours we choose. In keeping with the philosophy of H.A.G.S. with attitude as Seth Cohen says, 'it is above all about attitude'.

Our clothes will change as we get older as well and so they should. If like me you want to change your wardrobe as you need less business clothes and a more casual or personal persona, I highly recommend a personal dresser and/or coach, the service I offer my clients. We are in the position to help you reflect on your wardrobe and identify what remains relevant and what the gaps might be. We help you to explore ways in which to express yourself and your changing circumstances. You may very well want to communicate your identity rather than the business or corporate personality expected of you in your role as a business or professional woman. It's yet another opportunity to get creative.

It is time to give yourself permission to have fun with your clothes and accessories and discover what you want to communicate to the world about who you are. Apart from the latter, developing your own strong personal style means you do not have to change your wardrobe every season, saving money and the planet by not buying unnecessary items or garments you are unlikely to wear.

Every piece should count and contribute to the overall image you want to create. In doing so you stop being a slave to what the designers' vision of the style is for that season. You will develop your own timeless and unique image in colours and styles that suit you and communicates your unique personality. This is also the antidote to invisibility and more importantly, colluding with the anti-ageing mantra.

Although developing your own style should also be comfortable, it is absolutely not a license to become asexual and wearing shapeless clothing, drab colours with hair that has not seen a decent cut since your 40s. To top it all, a bland face with no makeup and colour. No wonder, women comment that they lose their confidence as they get older! Remember, grooming never goes out of fashion.

Despite popular belief, do not avoid colour. In fact, embrace colour wholeheartedly especially those that suit your skin tone. Take the time to have some fun with colour combinations, jewellery and glasses if you wear them. I managed to meet up with Tom Davies, designer of eyewear to the stars shared, who shared his words of wisdom with me as follows. The first thing we have to admit is that people often hate their own glasses. The reason we do may be down to the fact that not only do they not fit, slipping down the nose and leaving marks, but mainly because your glasses are often at odds with your own natural features with the result making you look less symmetrical. Symmetry is beauty!

It doesn't matter how old you are and who you are, glasses can and should be a positive part of your life. A great frame can give you confidence, even out asymmetrical features and add some colour to your life in the same way good makeup and clothes do. Most people like wearing sunglasses. Apart from being protective, they will equally even out your symmetry and are often designed in bolder colours and bolder lines. Think about buying your eyewear like sunglasses. You know you won't wear your sunglasses every day for two years. So, you tend to have a bit more fun with them. You don't need to spend a fortune on your glasses, but you do need more than two pairs. Ask yourself a valuation question. These glasses will define me. They will be on my face for years. Do I think one frame in brown is the way to go? No, you need a wardrobe of glasses. At least three pairs. Which you can accessorise with your outfits, with your life, with your occupation.

If you like to play tennis, should the glasses be the same ones you wear to work? If you are relaxing at home, should you have the same bold pair you like when you are out with your friends? Great eyewear can change your life. It's far too underrated by society. For something which everyone can see so clearly, defining your personality as well as how you look…logically, you start to realise that one pair for two years won't do. Love your glasses because you don't have to hate them!

Wise words which I have taken to heart since embracing the wearing of glasses and as Tom Davies advises, I have a few pairs of glasses to complement my outfits. I can truly say by changing my attitude towards wearing glasses and perceiving them as another fashion accessory, I no longer feel frumpy and advertising to the world that I am getting older. Instead, my attitude is, 'look at my great glasses!'

Let's also bust the final myth when it comes to the rules of society as far as older women are concerned. You do not have to cut your hair if you do not want to. There are endless examples of older women with gorgeous long grey locks. I think the aversion to long hair in older women go back to the stories and associations with wizened witches with wild hair and the derogatory labelling of older women as hags. The chapter on storytelling says more on this subject.

However, the key is to keep your crowning glory well-nourished and coiffed. Remember, grey is the new blond so embrace it without excuse or embarrassment, if you should choose not to colour your hair any longer. It is a personal choice and perhaps you may want to go pink, purple, green or any other colour to match your new style. We owe it to ourselves and younger women following on behind us to set an example of older women who refuse to become invisible and make that point on a daily basis in a colourful way. We have the power, let's use it to educate society and give other women the confidence to also express who they are.

In my previous life as an academic, I was greatly influenced by the philosophy of constructionism and discussed it in greater detail in the chapter on philosophy. In essence, it suggests that we collude with others and the world out there to create our experiences. Drawing inspiration from this philosophy, I know that we have the ability to create different experiences by actively and consciously making decisions and taking actions that will result in the outcomes we seek. Being invisible or not is, therefore, a choice we make and whichever one we choose will become our reality.

As you would have gathered by now, I feel passionate about our role and responsibility not to collude with the media and perpetuate the stereotypes of older women, subscribing to the anti-ageing rhetoric. Age is not a crime. We do not have to apologise for being a certain age or somehow perceive it as a personal failing. Nor is it a problem that needs to be solved with Botox, facelifts, creams and other expensive supernatural potions that will magically transport us back to a socially acceptable age.

However, we also don't have to look like our grandmothers! No disrespect to grandmothers. We lead very different lifestyles from those of our grandmothers and even our mothers. Most of us lead busy lives with women in their 70s and 80s continuing to work and/or run their own businesses. Read the story about Dilys, the oldest female and solo skydiver in the Guinee's Book of Records.

I strongly believe makeup is essential in making the most of our features in a natural way, unlike the plastered appearance women of the previous generation had to contend

166

with. The previous generation stayed away from adding colour to the wardrobe and played it safe with muted and dark colours. Makeup was rarely, if ever, applied. All adding to the invisibility issue we want to avoid. I have to thank my mother and her love of colour, which is probably why I have no qualms with wearing striking colours of shades that suit my colour palette.

As I have mentioned before, bold accessories and jewellery and scarfs are a must. Oh, and don't forget frumpy, lace-up shoes. Yuk! There are some very comfortable shoes available that are also very stylish, just shop around and yes, they may even lace-up, but using laces with attitude!

I reiterate clothes are so much more than merely covering our bodies and keeping us warm or cool. In a co-creative relationship with the designer, the wearer constructs a unique look that expresses her own personality and identity.

Looking good as older women do not require expensive designer clothes unless you can afford it. Furthermore, banish the erroneous belief that you have to select clothes to make you look younger or that being a certain age means you do not or should not care what you look like. Women need to celebrate their personal sense of style and expression no matter what their age.

Of course, clothes are only a small reflection of who we are, but research suggests that the clothes we wear can and do significantly impact our communication with others. Clothes allow us to consciously send out specific messages and thereby influence how we are perceived. How we feel about ourselves will determine the clothes we will wear and in turn affect the nature of our communication with others, not to mention our own sense of well-being and confidence.

I briefly introduced the inevitability of going grey above, a decision we all have to face at some stage. At the time of writing, I had an internal battle whether to allow my hair to go grey or continue to cover it up. I spent months researching the options of going grey. True to my personality, if I want something, I want it now. So, I engineered the acceleration of the process by, in my opinion, very successfully blending my own colour with that of my roots by using one of the many products available on greying the locks. If in doubt, consult a skilled hairdresser.

Being grey has certainly come a long way and as the younger generation would say, it is cool. I am stunned at how many young people actually choose to colour their hair grey. The decision to go grey can be quite liberating. No more trying to cover up the grey roots! For anyone not sure whether it is time to embrace the silver look, I recommend a tour of social media to help you realise how elegant and stylish grey can look, especially accompanied by the right clothes and accessories. Being grey is definitely not frumpy and it also does not mark a time for becoming colourless.

We of the older generation have the joy to get it for free and each one of us sporting our own unique shade of grey. I encourage you, therefore, to consider grey with a positive attitude and experiment until you find the colour combination that suits you and your personality.

However, having gone all out to give grey a go my training as an image consultant eventually made me realise that grey just doesn't suit a warm skinned autumn person like myself. I looked washed out and all my lovely autumn colours lost their sparkle. Unlike my mother who had very dark hair and eyes and whose greying hair was stunning, I inherited my father's reddish blond colouring. So, if you're unsure of whether to go grey or not, a consultation with a personal stylist or consultant can give you sound advice about colour and clothes as you get older. It may very well be time for a revamp of your wardrobe and hairstyle.

The Feather Makes the Bird

'When you don't dress like everybody else, you don't have to think like everybody else.'

– Iris Apfel

As you know by now, I believe that as older women, we have a responsibility to ensure that we do not collude with the myths of ageing and in particular, the image of what older women should look like. As there is a lot more about selecting our clothes, it will, therefore, be wise for us to give more thought to what and why we wear the particular items that we do.

My mother instilled in me a love of fashion and she was fond of saying that it is the feathers that make the bird. There is a myriad of reasons why we choose to wear what we do and it can range from pure practicalities of covering our bodies through to wearing clothes that epitomise our identity. Clothes have the ability to communicate much louder than words ever can when it comes to reflecting our unique personalities. We can be serious, successful, playful, naughty or anything else that takes our fancy and do so in style. It's not an either-or, we can do both.

Liz Clothier, a well-known stylist provided me with some suggestions of what we need to take into account when buying items of clothing to add or complement our wardrobe. 'Fashion is not frivolous. It is a part of being alive today.' This is a quote from Mary Quant, one of Liz' style heroes and an innovator of fashion as we know it today.

Liz swears by some well-chosen items such as:

Accessories

A scarf in the current season's colourway and print can be one of the best purchases you can make. It livens up a dull sweater, adds a pop of colour to a plain coat and acts as an extra layer when the temperature drops. There are always lots of lovely new prints and colours to choose from.

A bag is often a more expensive way to add a bit of current fashion trend to your look, but it doesn't have to be. There are lots of new shapes, fabrics and colours in most of the high street fashion retailers and if you just want to add a quick wardrobe update, then you don't have to spend a fortune. Unless you have lots of money to spend, her advice is to stick with more classic styles and colours if you're investing and 'go for the trend' if you're spending less.

A new pair of shoes can make you feel a million dollars or can result in pain! As we get older, we realise the benefits of a comfortable pair of shoes or boots. If you find a make that is really comfortable to you, then it's worth going back to the same brand when indulging your footwear fetish. Again, a pair of shoes can update a look by adding current colour, print and texture. Liz advises us to think carefully about what we will be wearing the shoes for. If it's a 'taxi to table' pair then go for it. However, if we're planning to wear them all day, most days then major on comfort. And a big tip: Never wear a new pair of shoes for an all-day city visit!

Other accessory options include belts, gloves, hats and jewellery. There are so many wonderful options and new looks available and it's a great way to update our style without breaking the bank or causing excess fashion anxiety!

Colour

The experience Liz has had of styling women from many different walks and times of life is that by the time we reach a certain age, we know what colours suit us. However, there's always an opportunity to experiment a little. Obviously, there are certain colours that suit us better than others, but that doesn't mean we can't experiment with different tones and combinations of the colours we love. Adding a new shade of colour can make us feel so much more 'on trend' and bring new life to an 'old favourite' garment.

As Chanel said: 'The best colour in the world is the one that looks best – on you!'

Fabrication

Every season, new treatment to fabrics emerge, often due to innovations in science and sourcing. Following the fashion-conscious theme, many fashion retailers are introducing ethically sourced clothing ranges and these are definitely worth looking out for. Recycled fabrics, new biodegradable yarns and fair-trade initiatives all play a major part in fashion today.

Leather and suede always make a big statement but we don't necessarily have to buy the real thing. There are many fashion-conscious alternatives, especially where suede-look fabrics are concerned. Velvet and jersey fabrics play a major part too and again, many are ethically sourced. Other fabric treatments come in the form of animal prints, checks and stripes. Adding a blouse in an animal print to a plain black trouser has an instant updating effect. And, if you're really daring, you could even try a pair of suedette or pleather trousers with a top you already own. There are so many options – it just takes a bit of experimentation.

I am also a passionate supporter of buying fewer but good quality clothes. Not only does this make sense for your budget, but it is also kind to the environment and the communities who create the products. Stylish clothes are not merely a frivolous indulgence, but it can benefit both you and the communities who have created and shared their unique heritage. In fact, this is a philosophy that extends to all aspects of my life from clothes, food, entertainment, holidays and everything else in between. As a previous chapter argues; quality over quantity.

A few good quality, classical pieces will not date and will always look good. I have some classical pieces that are over 20 years old. Maybe that is taking it to the extreme, but they still look good. As Liz suggests, accessories can transform your capsule wardrobe or those items you can't bear to part with.

At the time of writing, there is a big debate over the environmental costs of cheap clothing. Anyone with the slightest concern for the environment should consider carefully whether to contribute to the damage done to our beautiful but already overburdened planet. Less disposable and more quality clothing is much kinder to the environment as well as your wallet.

Then there is makeup and skincare to consider. So many of us when we reach a certain age give up on the use of makeup. Why, I fail to understand! Not only does makeup help give us confidence in our appearance, but it also allows us to enhance the attributes nature provided each one of us with, irrespective of age. Giving up on makeup colludes with the assumption that we become invisible beyond a certain age.

Some of you may find yourself in a rut with your makeup routine and not sure anymore as to how much or how little makeup you should wear and which colours are appropriate. Makeup provides us with the colour we need as we age. As we get older, our skin tones change as does the texture of our skin, making makeup even more important.

Some women feel subconscious wearing makeup after a certain age and often because of peer pressure from family and friends who think it is inappropriate for us as we get older; an assumption I passionately challenge! Makeup can work wonders in helping us make the most of our good features no matter how old we are.

We may also have become lazy and just wear any old thing as long as it is comfortable and over time the makeup regime becomes too much of bother as well. Fear not, because help is at hand in the form of a British based company that has developed a line of skincare and makeup for the older woman.

I introduced Tricia Cusden of Look Fabulous Forever in the chapter on gratitude.

Look Fabulous Forever is the success story of Tricia who started the company out of frustration due to the lack of awareness of the needs of the older skin by the beauty industry. Instead of retiring, she decided to start Looking Fabulous Forever. Having used a number of their products, including their skincare, I can highly recommend you give them a try. They ship their products around the world and you, therefore, don't need to be a resident in the U.K.

As a reminder, they have a significant amount of very useful tutorials on YouTube to give you advice on any aspect of skincare or makeup. It is worth a visit, especially if you've lost the will or know-how of applying makeup. There is no excuse for not taking care of yourself as doing so will significantly impact your self-confidence and sense of wellbeing.

Furthermore, we hugely underestimate the importance of colour in our mood and emotions. In the summer, we wake up and feel energised by the sun, the blue skies and the vibrancy of the summer flowers. In the U.K., given our rainfall, we have a lush, velvety green palette for the summer colours. Contrast that with the endless grey skies and hibernating plants and trees of the winter months. Which one resembles your wardrobe and then ask how does it impact your mood? If you feel you've become invisible, take a serious look at your wardrobe and it might give you the answer.

Just one scarf with colour or a colourful piece of jewellery and lippie will make all the difference. Whoever said we need to tone down colour as we get older needs a serious talking to. It is the time we need colour more than ever. We lose colour in our skin and our hair as we get older, so putting the colour back with makeup and clothes is paramount. Do yourself a favour and go on the many social platforms, search stylish older women and see the difference colour makes to their appearance. They are certainly not invisible and neither should you. Not to mention the benefits to your overall sense of wellbeing. It snowballs and impacts all aspects of your life. However, don't take my word for it, try it for yourself!

Returning to the message of this chapter, fashion is not merely a frivolous indulgence. It is a great source of personal expression and will go a long way to ensure that we do not disappear into oblivion. I reiterate that not taking care of our appearance means we collude with society and reinforce the negative stereotypes associated with older women. Furthermore, it is yet another example of the benefit we can gain from technology sitting in the comfort of our own homes.

Remember, the way we carry ourselves and wear what we wear communicates our unique brand to the world. As women, we know that appearance is incredibly powerful in sending out specific messages. Therefore, wear your clothes and accessories as an armour and a representation of your individuality and give others something to gossip about. As I will advocate throughout this book, it is even more pertinent as we get older.

So, be bold and choose the clothes and splash of makeup to celebrate your uniqueness, whatever your age. Go on and be a beautiful H.A.G. with attitude!

Women as Creators

'Why fit in when you were born to stand out!'

– Dr Seus

Most of us would give the answer to the question as to whether we are creative with an emphatic 'no'. However, each one of us has a creative side to our personalities irrespective of how we may choose to express our unique creativity.

It struck me when I reflected on discovering or rediscovering our creativity at a later stage in life that women are, in fact, the embodiment of creativity. Our bodies have been designed to materialise the ultimate form of creativity, namely to nurture and produce new life. How can we, therefore, say we are not creative?

If creativity is defined as the ability to create something unique and original then guess what, as women, we are creativity personified! Yet, many of us spend an inordinate amount of time and energy denying our creativity and ability to produce something new and novel. However, history is peppered with examples of women who have produced creative inventions that have benefitted society at large.

Observing children at play will confirm that as children, we possess an abundance of creativity and imagination. However, as we grow older, that creativity is more and more suppressed in favour of logic, reason, deadlines and have-to's and by the time we reach the world of work, it has almost been silenced completely.

Coupled with creativity is our inability to indulge in whatever takes our fancy, including doing absolutely nothing. We do not give ourselves permission to do or engage in activities that we consider frivolous and self-indulgent. Many of us have been exposed to a culture that advocates, nay insists, on delayed gratification; work before pleasure.

Doing absolutely nothing and indulging in time out allows the silenced, timid voice of creativity to once again emerge. As I reminded you in a previous chapter, our western culture values busyness and accomplishments over reflection and inactivity. We forget at the cost to our creativity and wellbeing that we are human 'beings' not human 'doings'.

Furthermore, the notion of having fun as an adult, particularly within the workplace, is an oxymoron. However, it is through fun and playfulness that we allow our creativity to surface. By the time we get to a certain age, we have forgotten what it is like to have fun. Once again, research reminds us that even as adults, it is through playfulness that we discover solutions and inspiration for new ideas.

There is not a shortage of advice on how to achieve and reacquaint ourselves with our creativity. The key thing is to find what works for you. However, the main ingredient is to bring a deep desire to do so on the journey of discovery.

One way is to revisit your childhood and remember the activities that brought you joy. How can you integrate some of these activities either into your careers or be enjoyed as hobbies now or when paid employment no longer features in your life? As your awareness grows so will your passion in these long-lost activities.

Above all, it is necessary to take a break from the perceived seriousness of business thinking. Take time out and spend it in nature, read, visit art galleries or listen to music and reignite those things that gave you so much joy as a child. Dare to be adventurous and stimulate your mind to remain open and nimble. Not only will you refresh your thinking and approach to your job, but it will help prepare you for a much more enjoyable life beyond employment.

The crux of it is that in order to enjoy ourselves and rediscover the pleasures gained through our creativity, we need to give ourselves permission to do so. Taking time to relax is a huge challenge for most of us. People may find that when they retire, they have difficulty in changing their lifestyle and discovering or rekindling pleasures in hobbies and new ways of being. As with any new skill learning to relax will feel uncomfortable in the beginning but with practise, it becomes easier.

Retirement is not about inactivity but instead, it is an opportunity to pursue a new purpose filled with those creative activities and hobbies we may not have had the time to do whilst in work. However, to get the most from your retirement requires planning and a conscious effort of redesigning the purpose of your life.

Find your passion and dust the cobwebs off your hidden dreams by grasping new opportunities or rediscovering long lost interests. Activity is the lifeblood of a fulfilled and meaningful life. Use all your experiences during your earlier years as a springboard for new expressions and interests. Not only will these activities guarantee a meaningful life, but they will ensure your brain is suitably exercised and stimulated.

I discussed at length in a previous chapter the need for living a purposeful life. Having a purpose is as important in later life as it was during the pursuit of a career. We all need to have something to get out of bed for in the morning and research suggests having a purpose contributes significantly to life expectancy. The scary thing is that you are now in charge of your purpose rather than abdicating it to the organisation to decide what your priorities should be. Our life takes on meaning through the quality of our experiences as well as activities with a purpose.

On the other hand, there are no deadlines in retirement. From personal experience, I can say that accepting this takes time. Don't stress about delays as these are no longer relevant or of any importance. As I mention on a number of occasions throughout the book, women are particularly skilled at feeling guilty about much of what they do or don't do. The dangers of guilt are something we might have to come to terms with when we retire or have more leisure time on our hands.

In the beginning, you may be racked with guilt that your days are not filled with to-do lists and chasing goals and objectives. It is, however, the time and opportunity to indulge in expressing our long-lost creativity in whatever form may be appropriate to us as individuals. Above all, make time to have fun!

Without jumping on my soapbox to argue that we live in a man's world created by men for men, we are socialised from a very early age to focus our attention on being pretty, nice, good girls. As we grow into women, we respond to the subtle messages that suggest women are the weaker and inferior sex and we fail to claim the same expectations set for men in terms of achievement.

Creativity is a highly sought-after commodity in business as it is the lifeblood of an organisation. Creative and innovative thinking is highly rewarded. There is also ample erroneous evidence to suggest that creativity is more likely to be associated with men than women. The result is that women will have less professional opportunities than men in an environment where creativity is highly prized.

Once again turning to science, research states that boys and girls are born with an equal amount of creative potential. In the UK a well-known television programme, *Horizon*, recently debated the controversial suggestion that men and women's brains are different. The findings were inconclusive with evidence to support both arguments.

However, what is important is our perceptions and how these will result in our view of reality, dictating our behaviour. Societal values and norms expect us as women to put the needs of others before our own and if we don't, we will eventually feel guilty and selfish for devoting time to develop our creativity at the expensive of nurturing others.

At some stage of our development, we are inspired by role models and supported by mentors, if we are lucky. Yet, there are fewer female role models for us to aspire to than the male role models available to boys. Instead, the media whose image of women is that of pretty, skinny supermodels or colourless, frumpy older women, constantly bombard women of all ages to conform to their expectation of what women should be and look like.

Young girls and women growing up need female role models and mentors to help them discover their worth and creativity. Those of us that have reached a certain age owe it to the younger generation to express and own our creativity. In doing so, it will give us the courage to act as mentors and role models to younger women who need the support and encouragement on their journey to discover their creativity.

One such role model that both inspired and moved me is the fairy story of success achieved by Susan Boyle. Apart from The Beatles and The Monkees, she is the only singer to have simultaneously topped the music charts in both the U.K. and U.S.A. on two occasions in one year. Yet her success is permeated by gratitude for the career she has enjoyed in later life. The song that catapulted her onto the musical scene, *I Dreamt a Dream* from Les Misérables, will for me always be associated with Susan Boyle.

She has gone from strength to strength with a string of achievements under her belt. Growing up she never wavered in her passion for singing despite having her share of challenges throughout life, including being diagnosed with Asperger's syndrome. Now at 58, she expressed an interest in pursuing the necessary training to turn her hand to opera. What a wonderful role model for all of us over the 50s who think it is too late to pursue our interests and dreams. She is also a beautiful mature woman who expresses her unique beauty. I am reminded by another famous singer, Adelle when being taken to task for her larger size commented that she 'makes music for ears and not eyes'. Well said!

My challenge, therefore, to all women out there and particular those, who like me have more time to nurture and express their brand of creativity, we owe it to the younger women growing up now. Claim your worth and be an inspirational role model that girls and younger women can aspire to. I once again remind you that age is no barrier to creativity!

The Art of Dying

'Death is the final stage of growth.'

– Elisabeth Kübler-Ross

Some may consider it strange that I've included a chapter on dying when the book is relentlessly devoted to living with the right attitude and to celebrate every day we have. However, dying is a natural part of living and at some stage, it comes to us all.

Many of us grow older either dreading our mortality or wrapping ourselves in denial of the fact that it is an intimate companion of life. However, ageing is erroneously associated with the end of life. We speak of death and ageing in the same breath, but they should not be confused with one another. Coming to terms with our mortality frees us to enjoy and make the most of each moment we are alive.

Sadly, in Western cultures, in particular, discussions regarding death and dying are avoided at all costs or sidestepped with intricate footwork that any dancer will envy. However, breaking the silence allows us and our loved ones to plan for the inevitable ensuring the appropriate care and support is available when needed.

My brother's journey with terminal cancer and the importance to him and his partner to plan the end provided great comfort to them both. We should not wait until the end comes towards us with great speed. Instead, a good death starts with a good life and living each day with meaning and gratitude for the small but important things and a sense of living with purpose.

My husband frequently laments the fact that he will not enjoy all the marvels of technology yet to come. On the other hand, he mourns the perceived romantic simplicity of the 'good old days.' Montaigne captures this paradox in his magnificent meditation on death and the art of living by saying: 'To lament that we shall not be alive a hundred years hence, is the same folly as to be sorry we were not alive a hundred years ago.'

If we think about it, every day we wake up a slightly different person. Each day a small part of us dies and changes, so why perceive death as one major event in the distant future when it comes every day in one way or another. It is worth reminding ourselves that as soon as we are born, the ageing process begins, taking us one step closer to death.

Acknowledging and accepting the inevitability of our mortality bestows on us the gift of passionately living in the present. Each one of us will choose to spend our lives in different ways and accepting the experiences and circumstances put in our path. We may share our lives with a loved one, enjoy the peace of solitude, marvelling at the wonders of nature, engaged in a favourite activity or simply getting on with life.

Sometimes those who fear death the most are often the ones who have not really lived or are burdened with unfulfilled dreams, unresolved issues or allowed life to pass them by. Death provides a context for life and a reminder that life should be meaningful, whatever our personal definition of a meaningful life might be. Furthermore, each one of us will find the solace needed to make sense not only of death but life as well. For some, it is a religious belief, for others a spiritual way of being, embracing an eclectic set of beliefs, whilst others bow to the hand of fate. Whatever and wherever we draw our support from, it will offer comfort to us throughout life, including the final moments.

We have all had and will continue to have, experiences with death. These experiences are unique to us all and will determine what our attitude is likely to be towards death. If our experiences are of a loved one having lived a long, healthy life ending with a peaceful death, then it will no doubt be more positive than having a loved one torn from life violently or at a young age.

Such an experience makes it much more difficult to come to terms with death. The unexpected, brutal death of my eldest brother changed the perception of life, living and death that remained with my parents until the end. On the other hand, the death of my younger brother was different.

His journey with terminal cancer and his decision to eventually cease treatment meant he took charge of his death, giving him a sense of agency. He embodied the philosophy of living for each moment as if it was his last, which eventually, as for all of us, it was. His journey made me realise that death, as with birth, is only a very brief stage of life. Our focus should, therefore, be on the life between these two bookends.

The ebb and flow of life are marked by a number of stages with the preceding one giving way to the next. Each one of life's stages brings with it its own gift and it is for us to both recognise and treasure these gifts. At some stage of our lives, we will look back and begin to understand how the stages fit together and understand the purpose of our personal journeys.

In order to benefit from the stages of life, we have to accept the limitations of each stage and move on to the next when the time comes. Each stage offers us the opportunity to develop a flow of life and learning to successfully navigate the ever-changing currents of life. Some of us may get stuck in a particular stage and some may skip a stage altogether, not always of our own doing but determined by traumatic external events.

The purpose of our initial stage in life is to learn how to adapt to others in society and become aware of the rules of behaviour within our respective cultures. We do this by mimicking others around us. Navigating this stage successfully results in us becoming self-sufficient and autonomous human beings.

Failing to transition from this stage to the next will result in us forever trying to please everyone else at the expense of pursuing what we want in life. We may go to great pains to avoid being judged by others and to gain their approval. It may also delay the process of getting to know who we are and what makes us tick as an individual. The challenge is to become integrated into our respective communities whilst at the same time express our unique talents and personalities.

Oh, for the passion of adolescence! It bursts forth marking this stage one of self-discovery through experimentation and curiosity. The world is our oyster and adventures beckon. We undergo significant transformation both physically and emotionally. It is the phase when we challenge family ideas and pushing the boundaries of both family as well as institutional customs and ideologies. Instead, we may align ourselves with the social, political and religious causes that resonate with our emerging values and beliefs. The challenge is to maintain a balance between developing independence whilst at the same time remain rooted in the support offered by our family and culture.

We go into the world to leave our mark through the education and experiences we choose to pursue. It is during this stage that we develop the courage to discover who we are and what separates us from others. We now begin to establish our personal boundaries to empower us to reject the values and beliefs that are incongruent with our own. We experiment with things, make mistakes and hopefully learn from them, whilst continuing to develop.

It is an exciting stage of discovery and may very well be the reason why some people get stuck in this stage and struggle to let go and embrace the next phase of the journey. The need to constantly seek the thrill of exploration and adventure may lead to a reluctance to accept that all endeavours will eventually end.

Coupled with this phase of adventure is the recognition and acceptance of our limitations. Being confronted by our failures is part of the journey of personal growth. If successful, we gain insight and acceptance that we cannot pursue everything. We have to be selective and focus on the important activities we want to spend our precious time on.

The stage of maturity is marked by consolidation and embracing our individual potential. It is a significant stage in our adult lives and with the onset of midlife, we begin to contemplate the true meaning of our individual lives. It is the stage when we develop a deeper understanding not only of what it means to be human but more importantly what it means to be you. On the other hand, some might find themselves in an existential crisis also, which has been associated with the midlife crisis. Although, in another chapter, I spent time exploring and challenging some of the assumptions associated with the midlife crisis.

Then follows the time to de-clutter our lives, ridding ourselves of time-wasting activities and energy-draining relationships. We may also start making significant changes in our lives as we recognise what is of importance to us. The result is that we nurture and treasure the activities and people that truly matter to us. In essence, it is about creating the legacy we will leave behind.

Leaving this stage for the next means letting go of the urgency to continuously achieve and master the next challenge or goal. Some of us may struggle to accept that it is impossible to achieve everything we desire nor would we have the energy to constantly pursue elusive goals and the need to accumulate ever more things, status or power.

With a bit of luck, we move into the stage of wisdom and benevolence. It is a time when we can make significant contributions to society. This is also the stage in life when we come to terms with our mortality. It is in my opinion the stage when it all comes together and we are able to enjoy the fruits of our labour. It is also the time when we pass on the wisdom we have gathered through the journey of our life. It is time to become important volunteers and mentors to the younger generation.

Age is marked by a lengthy accumulation of knowledge and experience out of which hopefully wisdom may grow. Some cultures recognise the value and benefit the older generation has to offer society. Alas, in other societies, especially the West, the older generation are often ignored or discarded and forgotten.

This time of wisdom and contemplation is when we decide what it was all about. Taking the time to reflect on what the purpose of our lives was and the legacy we want to leave behind will help us to make the most of the final stage of our lives.

My younger brother, Eugene or Duimpie as he was affectionately known and his philosophy of life meant he insisted that life was for the living and that Pieter, his partner, should get on with life after he was gone. My brother had the wisdom to recognise that a surviving partner may often suffer from survivors' guilt. Easy to say, I know, but hopefully, in time we will come to treasure our memories and be grateful for every day we've been given and make the most of it. We will follow our loved ones soon enough.

So, despite the inevitable, we must get our priorities in order and focus on the life we have yet to live before the final moment arrives. Thanks to modern technology, medicine and changes in mindset, life after 50 has a great deal to offer. No doubt the average lifespan will continue to be extended as a result. I hope what this book has gone some way in achieving is that you will not see the midlife as being about reclaiming your lost youth but instead being about planning how to live the next half of your life.

Death is not an enemy to be feared or defeated. Instead, it gives meaning to our lives. It urges us to do something worthwhile with the life we have while we have it. It is up to us to live that life in a way that is fulfilling and rewarding. It is not about the length of time, but the quality of a life well-lived!

"You can't go back and change the beginning but you can start where you are and change the ending."

– Author Unknown

Conclusion

It is with reluctance that I draw the research and writing of my book to a conclusion. There is still so much out there to discover and share with you all, but if I don't stop, this book will never see the light of day. Hopefully, I have given you enough inspiration and encouragement to go out and explore the areas you would like to know more about or expand your knowledge and understanding.

I am sure that on more than one occasion, you have rejected my advice or musings. I hope that in time, you will reconsider and reflect on what these words may convey to you and your life. Coming back to parts of the book may very well give you a new perspective or even an aha moment.

There is an endless flow of encouraging stories of ordinary men and women who do amazing things at advanced years. I have shared a number of those with you throughout the book. All we have to do is look for them and as role models, they encourage us to start small and build on the first few steps to a different and more positive outlook to getting older.

As most of us will live 20 or 30 years beyond the official retirement age instead of winding down it is time for renewal. We are probably the first of a generation that is likely to live well into their 80s, 90s and even become centenaries. Remember the world doesn't care whether we stay up to date with changes or not. It will keep on turning and it is up to us to adapt and adopt different ways and lead a fulfilling and exciting life or instead, become a grump and a dinosaur.

Remain young at heart by challenging yourself and take risks, no matter how small. It helps us to rewire the brain. Be bold and be brave! Take responsibility for your own life and live it to the full. We owe it to ourselves and to embrace life with resilience, a positive attitude, whatever challenges cross our paths.

We are setting an example for the younger generation that getting older does not equate to decline and inevitable ill health. Through our lifestyle choices and attitude, we can demonstrate to the next generation that getting older offers many advantages to further express one's individuality and that leading a full life is a choice available to us all irrespective of age.

Furthermore, I encourage you to recognise our responsibility to be role models for the next generation of older women to follow. It is not just for us, but we are the trailblazers and owe it to the next generation to demonstrate that there is life beyond 50. I once again remind you that there are no rules to ageing. You make and decide the rules that suit you and to hell with everyone else!

Let us together break the erroneous mould associated with older women and instead live lives that are examples of the joys and rewards the second half of life has to offer. It is our gift to society and we are probably the first generation to embrace an alternative belief that more accurately reflects the reality of being an older woman. Especially a H.A.G.S. with attitude!

References

Applewhite, A. (2019). *This Chair Rocks: A Manifesto Against Ageism*, London: Melville House

Boone, J., Matz-Costa, C., Smyer, M. A. (2016). Retirement Security: It's Not Just About the Money, *American Psychology, 71(4):334-44*

Bradley Hagerty, B. (2016). *Life Reimagined: The Science, Art, and Opportunity of Midlife*, New York, N. Y.: Riverhead Books

Cavendish, C. (2019). *Extra Time: Ten Lessons for an Ageing World,* London: Harper Collins Publishers

Cohen, A.S., (2012) *Advanced Style*, New York, N.Y. Penguin Random House Group

Diaz, C and Bark, S. (2016). *The Longevity Book*, U.S.A.: Harper Wave

Chopra, D. (1993). *Ageless Body, Timeless Mind*: *A Practical Alternative to Growing Old*, London: Ryder

Earle, L. (2018). *The Good Menopause Guide*, London: Orion Publishing Company

Hollis, J. (2005). *Finding Meaning in the Second Half of Life*, New York, N. Y.: Gotham Books

Huffpost.com

Leider, R. J. (2015). *The Power of Purpose* (3rd Ed.), CA. U.S.A.: Berrett-Koehler Publishers, Inc.

Lookingfabulousforever.com

Low, G., Molzahn, A. E., Schopflocher, D. (2013). Attitudes to aging mediate the relationship between older peoples' subjective health and quality of life in 20 countries, *Health Quality and Life Outcomes, 11:146*

Modernelderacademy.com

Nelson, T. D. (2016). Promoting Healthy Aging by Confronting Ageism, *American Psychologist, 71(4):334-344*

Northrup, C. (2012). *The Wisdom of Menopause*, New York, N.Y.: Bantam Books.

Northrup, C. (2010). *Women's Bodies, Women's Wisdom*, New York, N. Y.: Bantam Books.

Robertson, D. A., Weiss, D. (2017). In the Eye of the Beholder: Can Counter-Stereotypes Change Perceptions of Older Adults' Social Status? *Psychology and Aging, 32(6):531-542*

Smedley, K. (2013) *Live the Life You Love at 50+*, England: McGraw-Hill Education

Shultz, K. S. (2015). *Retirement the Psychology of Reinvention: A Practical Guide to Planning and Enjoying the Retirement You've Earned*, New York, N.Y.: DK Publishing.

Silversurfers.com

Stewart, S. A. (2018). *Winter's Graces: The Surprising Gifts of Later Life*, U.S.A. She Writes Press

Taosinstitute.net

Thomas M. Hess, T. M., O'Brien, E.L., Kornadt, A. E., Fung, H. H., Voss, P. Rothermund, K. and Popham, L. E., (2017). Context Influences on the Relationship Between Views of Aging and Subjective Age: The Moderating Role of Culture and Domain of Functioning, *Psychology and Aging*, *32(5):419-431*

Voss, P. Kornadt, A. E., Rothermund, K. (2017). Getting What You Expect? Future Self-Views Predict the Valence of Life Events, *Developmental Psychology, 53(3):567-580*

Walker, B. G. (1985). *The Crone: Woman of Age, Wisdom, and Power*, New York, N. Y.: Harper One

Waxman, B. (2016). *The Middlescence Manifesto: Igniting the Passion of Midlife*, CA, U.S.A.: Barbara Waxman

Weareageist.com